AF713223

HIV/AIDS and Food and Nutrition Security

From Evidence to Action

Stuart Gillespie
and
Suneetha Kadiyala

Food Policy Review 7

International Food Policy Research Institute
2033 K Street, N.W.
Washington, D.C.

International Food Policy Research Institute
2033 K Street, NW
Washington, DC 20006-1002 USA
Telephone +1-202-862-5600
www.ifpri.org

Library of Congress Cataloging-in-Publication Data

Gillespie, Stuart.
HIV/AIDS, food and nutrition security : from evidence to action / Stuart Gillespie and Suneetha Kadiyala.
p. cm. — (Food policy review ; 7)
Includes bibliographical references.
ISBN 0-89629-506-0 (alk. paper)
1. AIDS (Disease). 2. HIV infections. 3. Nutrition—Evaluation. 4. Nutrition policy. 5. Food—Safety measures. 6. World health. I. Kadiyala, Suneetha. II. Title. III. Series.
RA643.8.G535 2005
616.97′920654—dc22 2005003712

Contents

Tables

Figures

Boxes

Foreword

The HIV/AIDS pandemic is a global crisis with consequences that will be felt for decades to come. The ability of households and communities to ensure their food and nutrition security in the face of AIDS is being severely challenged. Livelihoods are being eroded through the effects of premature illness and death on household labor power and through the fracturing of intergenerational knowledge transfer. Social relations and capacity to care are being put under immense strain by HIV-related stigma and exclusion, increasing orphaning rates, and reduced incentives for collective action. Financial stress is increased as expenditures for health care and funerals increase, and as credit becomes harder to access. Labor losses affect the ability to farm and to maintain common property resources, and assets are sold off to raise cash. Though sub-Saharan Africa is currently being hit hardest, the spread of HIV in other regions, especially South Asia, is accelerating, and the downstream impacts are beginning to be felt.

The effects are two-way. Not only does HIV/AIDS precipitate and exacerbate food and nutrition insecurity, but the spread of the virus is accelerated when people—because of their worsening poverty—are forced to adopt ever more risky food provisioning strategies.

This review is the most comprehensive of its kind to date. Drawing on a detailed evidence base of over 150 studies encompassing various disciplines (including nutrition, economics, epidemiology, and sociology), it builds a picture of what is known about the interactions between HIV/AIDS and food and nutrition security, and what this knowledge implies for food- and nutrition-relevant policy. Summaries of all studies are provided in annexes for easy reference.

Three maps are used to navigate this new universe. The first map depicts interactions at a societal level, showing the waves of determinants of HIV infection, from macro to micro levels, and the subsequent waves of AIDS impacts, rippling out from micro to macro levels. The second map focuses on household and community interactions—again showing how HIV/AIDS affects, and is affected by, different livelihoods. And the third map shows the interactions at the level of an individual person, highlighting the critical importance of nutritional status.

The authors use these three maps to structure their review of the evidence. First they examine evidence regarding the interactions between HIV/AIDS and food and nutrition security, and then review the recent attempts by different stakeholders to respond to these interactions. The final section addresses the particular challenges of scaling up, mainstreaming, and capacity development. Responses need to be scaled up, geographically and organizationally, to match the scale, breadth, and interconnectedness of the pandemic's causes and impacts. The authors prescribe the use of an adaptable "HIV/AIDS lens" to literally re-view existing policies and programs from the perspective of what HIV/AIDS is doing to them.

The review will serve as a valuable resource for institutions struggling to confront the implications of HIV/AIDS for food and nutrition-relevant policies and programs, and for IFPRI and its partners as we further focus on research issues that promise positive impacts for people affected by HIV/AIDS.

Joachim von Braun
Director General, IFPRI

Acknowledgments

We are indebted to members of the Regional Network on HIV/AIDS, Rural Livelihoods and Food Security (RENEWAL), especially Michael Loevinsohn, for numerous insights gleaned over the last few years. We also thank Tony Barnett, Hans Binswanger, Joan Holmes, Peter Matlon, Roy Stacy, Alan Whiteside, an anonymous reviewer, and participants at the June 2004 seminar at IFPRI for comments made on an earlier draft. We thank IFPRI's Publication Review Committee for shepherding this review to the publication stage and Betsy Finley and Ginette Mignot for help in finalizing the document. Finally, we are very grateful to the United States Agency for International Development, the World Food Programme, the United Nations Development Programme, and the Millennium Project Hunger Task Force for funding this work.

Introduction

The HIV/AIDS pandemic is a global crisis with impacts that will be felt for decades to come. More than 20 million people have died since the first case was reported in 1981. In 2004, HIV/AIDS killed more than 3 million people, and nearly 5 million became infected, bringing to 39 million the number of people living with the virus around the world. More than 25 million of these people live in sub-Saharan Africa, where in some countries one in three adults is infected. In sub-Saharan Africa, more than 12 million children have lost one or both parents to AIDS (UNAIDS/WHO 2004).

The situation is also becoming increasingly serious in other parts of the world, notably Central and South Asia. By the end of 2003, over 5 million people in India alone were estimated to be living with HIV/AIDS (UNAIDS/WHO 2004). Recognizing that large-scale preventive action is urgently required in these countries, much of this review focuses on the situation in sub-Saharan Africa, where the food and nutrition security impacts are most serious and where there is more experience to build on. We do, however, include a case study of India, highlighting the fertile terrain for the spread and impacts of HIV/AIDS on the subcontinent.

HIV/AIDS is a long-wave crisis, but it is made up of several waves (Barnett and Whiteside 2002). The first is the wave of HIV infection; the second is a wave of opportunistic infections, the most common being tuberculosis. This is followed, after a three- to eight-year lag, by the third wave, consisting of AIDS illness and death. The fourth and last is the wave of impacts on households, communities, and nations.

A few countries are now over the peak of the first wave, such as Uganda, Senegal, Thailand, and Brazil. But no country has yet reached the crest of the third wave, and for the majority of affected countries the fourth wave is only just beginning. This fourth wave, which may include social and political destabilization, will engulf countries for decades to come and demand massive responses.

Such responses need to continue to be grounded in the three fundamental principles of prevention, care and treatment, and mitigation, but they must also take into account the integral role of food and nutrition. These responses also need to be far more broadly based and better connected to match the scale, breadth, and interconnectedness of the pandemic's causes and impacts.

We do not know how severe the impacts of the third and fourth waves will be: little about this pandemic is linear, and AIDS is a unique threat (see Box 1). What, for example, will be the likely long-term damage—social, economic, and psychological—wrought by the orphaning of millions of children? We do know that impacts will continue to be felt for years to come, and the situation will get significantly worse before it gets better. Against this backdrop, it is clear that whatever the effectiveness of the highly publicized but slow-moving roll-out of antiretroviral therapy, a much larger and more comprehensive response is needed from many quarters.

This is the stark challenge we face. The good news is that our understanding of the dynamics of HIV epidemics and their multidimensional effects is improving, and awareness is growing of the need for development policy and practice to be more responsive to the HIV/AIDS crisis. This shift derives not only from the worsening and increasingly visible impacts of AIDS but also from the realization that original sectoral objectives are unlikely to be achieved without such a proactive stance: the Millennium Development Goals (MDGs) for Africa, for example, will not be achieved without a comprehensive response to HIV epidemics. We are at last beginning to see real, practical action in some of these areas.

One major group of impacts of HIV/AIDS relates to the ability of households and communities to ensure food and nutrition security. In this book we highlight the main interactions between HIV/AIDS and food and nutrition insecurity and suggest effective responses. An earlier paper by one of the authors (Loevinsohn and Gillespie 2003a) proposed a framework to facilitate a more holistic understanding of these interactions and ultimately to improve the means of responding at different levels. This review intends to put flesh on this framework as evidence continues to emerge both of the impacts and (albeit more slowly) of effective solutions. The review thus has the following objectives:

1. Demonstrate the need to take a fully comprehensive and holistic approach to investigating how HIV/AIDS is affecting (and affected by) people, communities, and governments, in order to better understand the various risks, impacts, and responses.
2. Review the evidence behind the "upstream" factors and processes that contribute

Box 1. Why AIDS is unique

- It is incurable and fatal.
- It kills the most productive members of society and kills them slowly, drawing others from the workforce to care for those who are sick.
- Life-prolonging treatment will remain inaccessible for the vast majority of people living with HIV/AIDS.
- It is socially invisible and mired in silence and stigma.
- It is a long-wave crisis with a very long incubation period between infection and full-blown symptoms, during which individuals are infective; and invisibility and long duration combine to increase chances of HIV transmission.
- It has both rural and urban dimensions and significant urban-rural linkages.
- It affects both the rich and the poor, though the poor are most severely exposed.
- It affects both sexes but is not gender-neutral: women are physiologically, economically, and culturally more at risk of HIV infection and AIDS.
- Just as its impacts intensify, with a parallel need for action, the actual *capacity to act* is declining precipitously. The United Nations has recently drawn attention to the "triple threat" of food insecurity, AIDS, and deteriorating capacity (UN 2004).

Adapted from Haddad and Gillespie 2001.

to HIV spread as well as the various "downstream" impacts of AIDS and premature death.

3. Review the responses to these risks and impacts at different levels, from individuals and households up to national governments, along with the implications for international agencies.

Defining Concepts and Mapping Interactions

Food security here refers to physical and economic access to food of sufficient quality and quantity. Food security is necessary, but of itself insufficient, for ensuring nutrition security. *Nutrition security* is achieved for a household when secure access to food is coupled with a sanitary environment, adequate health services, and adequate care to ensure a healthy life for all household members. *Hunger*[1] is another

[1]The hungry are a subset of the food-insecure, who in turn are a subset of the nutrition-insecure. Some of the food-insecure are not currently hungry, although they are at risk of becoming so because of their uncertain access to food. Moreover, some of the nutrition-insecure are not food-insecure, as their condition may result from deficits in the health- and care-related determinants of nutrition security.

related term, but because food-provisioning capacities are being undermined in ways that may not yet be manifest as hunger, we focus here on the broader concepts of food and nutrition security.

HIV/AIDS and food and nutrition insecurity are becoming increasingly entwined in a vicious cycle, with food insecurity heightening *susceptibility* to HIV exposure and infection, and HIV/AIDS in turn heightening *vulnerability* to food insecurity (Loevinsohn and Gillespie 2003a). To better understand these interactions at different levels so that they may be effectively addressed, we need to map them.

Three useful maps can be drawn, corresponding to the different levels of interaction. First, societal-level interactions can be represented by Figure 1, which, from left to right, shows the waves of determinants of HIV infection from macro to micro levels, and the subsequent waves of impacts from micro to macro.

The top left quadrant shows various factors that condition *susceptibility* to the HIV virus at different levels. Susceptibility has two components:

- the chance of being *exposed* to the virus, which in turn relates to a person's risk environment and the *riskiness* of her/his behaviors (both of which may be related), and
- the chance of being *infected* with the virus once exposed.

Resistance is the ability of an individual to proactively avoid infection by HIV. Some of the main strategies for promoting resistance can be seen in the bottom left quadrant.

The epicenter of Figure 1 is HIV infection in an individual. Following HIV infection, we can see in the top right quadrant the various sources and levels of *vulnerability* to AIDS-related impacts. These impacts are not one-time events but processes, often hidden and gradual but potentially very destructive. *Resilience* bears a similar relation to vulnerability as resistance does to susceptibility: it refers in particular to the active responses (shown in the bottom right quadrant) that enable people to avoid the worst consequences of AIDS at different levels, or to recover faster to a level accepted as normal (Loevinsohn and Gillespie 2003a).

A vicious cycle begins when impact waves later become causal waves. One extreme example is transactional sex. Because of her husband's illness or death from AIDS, a woman may be forced to trade sex for cash to feed her children. By doing so she drastically increases the risk of becoming infected herself. Thus some of the main impacts may also themselves increase risk, and some of the main mitigation responses may also *prevent* future infection.

The second map (Figure 2) focuses on the level of household and community interactions, again showing susceptibility and vulnerability forming a cycle. In a sense this map is an elaboration of the dynamics at the micro and meso levels of Figure 1.

Figure 1 HIV/AIDS determinants, impacts, and responses

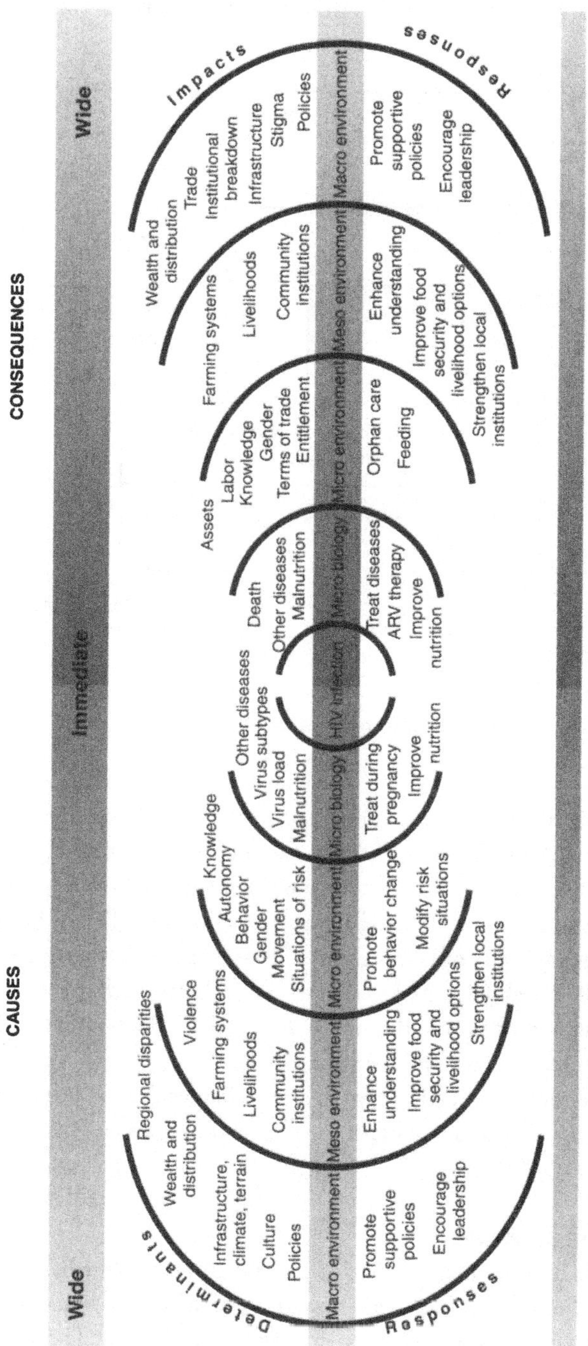

Source: Loevinsohn and Gillespie 2003a.

Figure 2 Understanding HIV/AIDS in the context of people's livelihoods

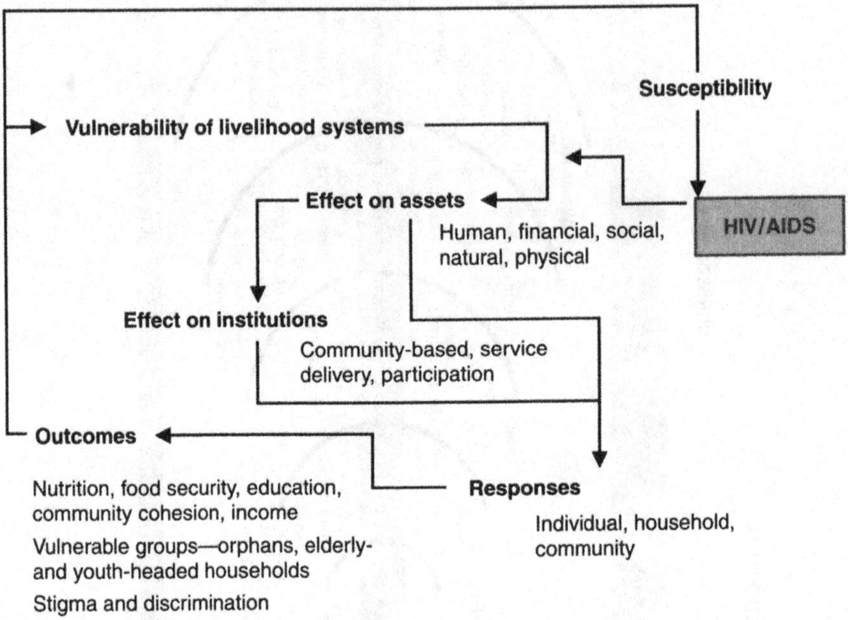

Source: Adapted from TANGO International 2002.

It is essentially an adaptation of the Sustainable Livelihoods framework (Carney 1998), which shows how HIV/AIDS affects, and is affected by, livelihoods. The risks people face of contracting HIV will be governed partly by the susceptibility of the livelihood system on which they depend. The effect of HIV/AIDS on assets and institutions is a measure of vulnerability. These effects will determine the strategic responses that households adopt to deal with this threat. Such responses in turn will have outcomes—nutrition and food security among them—that will themselves condition future susceptibility and vulnerability.

The third map (Figure 3), shown in a later chapter, shows the interactions at the level of the individual and highlights the critical importance of nutritional status.

The Evidence Base

Though it has been agonizingly slow to take off and there remain significant biases and gaps, the literature in this area is now growing rapidly. A detailed evidence base, including over 150 studies, has been annexed to this review. The vast majority of these studies are peer-reviewed journal articles or reports, most of which have been written during the last five years. Many are still in the form of working papers (for example, Ainsworth and Semali 2000, Gertler et al. 2003, and Mather et al. 2004a) but make important new contributions to the literature.

Socioeconomic impact studies range from those employing rigorous quantitative methodologies (for example, studies by Mather et al. 2004b, Deininger et al. 2003, and Mason et al. 2003) or qualitative methodologies (such as Barnett and Blaikie 1992, Barnett et al. 1995, and Rugalema 1999) to cross-sectional descriptive analyses (including Shah et al. 2001, SADC FANR 2003, and Drimie 2003) to some that are almost anecdotal. The last are not included in this evidence base.

Descriptive studies provide suggestive evidence of impacts (among them Mutangadura 2000, Tibaijuka 1997, and Gilborn et al. 2001), whereas larger household surveys that test hypotheses (such as Gertler et al. 2003 and studies by Michigan State University) provide further evidence. Many studies have been conducted in regions of high HIV prevalence, such as Rakai district in Uganda (see Menon et al. 1998; Barnett and Blaikie 1992) and Kagera in Tanzania (see Ainsworth and Semali 2000; Beegle 2003; Lundberg and Over 2000). The cumulative results of these studies help us build up a picture of dynamics and impacts. But caution is required to avoid unwarranted generalizations: the more we learn about interactions and responses, the more we understand how context-specific many of them are. Little investment has been made to revisit these sites in order to monitor changes over time. The RENEWAL initiative is engaged in one such study in Zambia, and Michigan State University, with its partners in Kenya, Malawi, Mozambique, Rwanda, and Zambia, is conducting nationally representative panel surveys to study the long-term impact of adult mortality (Mather et al. 2004b).

There are other assessment challenges. Ethical considerations often preclude direct comparisons of AIDS-related and non-AIDS-related deaths. Menon et al. (1998), Janjaroen et al. (1998), Bechu (1998), Urassa et al. (2001), Morris et al. (2000), Rugalema et al. (1999), and Fox et al. (2004) are important examples of studies that directly compare the impact of AIDS deaths with deaths from other causes. Many studies have used proxy indicators, such as chronic illness or the number of orphans, to compare AIDS-affected and unaffected households (FASAZ/FAO 2003; SADC FANR 2003; studies by Michigan State University). The use of these proxies has certain limitations: *illness,* for example, can range from complete debility to not feeling well. Mather et al. (2004b) provide convincing analysis of the strong contribution of AIDS to prime-age adult mortality in high-prevalence countries such as Kenya, Malawi, and Zambia. Innovative ways of assessing the effects of HIV/AIDS continue to emerge: Gertler et al. (2003), for example, use self-reported ability to perform activities of daily living to measure chronic illness. Indicators of "affectedness," such as various so-called coping strategies, may be problematic. By the time such indicators become significant, the household may already be deeply affected by the epidemic, and these responses may be quite different from earlier ones.

That the unit of analysis of most studies is the household is itself problematic. As Barnett and Whiteside (2002) note, households that dissolve or disappear, arguably the most severely affected, are lost to research. Household-level analyses also fail to capture the complex interactions and relations between and within households, household clusters, and communities. Other studies employing methods and tools from disciplines such as sociology, political science, and anthropology are clearly needed to refine our understanding of, for example, the complex interactions between households and communities, issues of power, and capacity to respond at various levels.

Part 1

Interactions

In Part 1, we review current evidence for the different interactions between HIV/AIDS and food and nutrition security. We begin by examining interactions that condition susceptibility to HIV infection and then review the more highly developed literature on the downstream impacts of HIV/AIDS on individuals, households, and communities. The structural logic derives from Figure 1, reading from left to right.

Chapter 1

Impacts of Food and Nutrition Insecurity on the Spread of HIV

The microbe is nothing, the terrain everything.
—Louis Pasteur, 1860

HIV epidemics are environmentally driven. Pasteur's observation succinctly captures the power of environment, which encompasses everything from the microbiological environment represented by a person's nutritional and health status to the macroenvironmental level of policy, culture, and economy (see Figure 1). We have known for 20 years what causes HIV infection, but we are only now beginning to understand what fuels HIV epidemics. The use of the term *pandemic* conceals the fact that multiple epidemics may differ in causation, velocity, duration, and impact. These epidemics are endogenous to livelihood systems and fundamentally shaped by existing socioeconomic and cultural systems and conditions (Loevinsohn and Gillespie 2003a; Barnett and Whiteside 2002). Understanding of the driving forces behind HIV infection—the socioeconomic factors that condition behaviors, along with the biological factors that determine an individual's susceptibility or resistance—is now growing.

Food insecurity and malnutrition may accelerate the spread of HIV, both by increasing people's exposure to the virus and by increasing the risk of infection following exposure:

- *Exposure.* Poverty and food insecurity may place people in situations of heightened risk of exposure to the virus. Because they are food-insecure, people may be less able to access information about HIV/AIDS or less able to act on their knowledge of risk to minimize HIV exposure. They may be forced to separate from their families to earn a livelihood. Women may be forced into transactional sex in order to feed their families.

- *Transmission/infection.* Food insecurity, along with poor health and care, may lead to increased malnutrition rates. Malnutrition in turn may lead to increased HIV transmission efficiency by lowering immunity and compromising gut and genital mucosal integrity. Malnutrition among pregnant and lactating women may increase vertical transmission rates. The next section highlights the existing evidence for these two statements.

Food Insecurity and Exposure to HIV

In fact it is hunger that is leading to the rise in HIV infections in this area.
—Religious leader in Vizimba, Malawi, focus group, quoted in Bryceson et al. 2004

Few studies have rigorously investigated the direct impact of food insecurity on the adoption of high-risk behaviors. Those that have done so use a poverty/equity lens to view the risk of exposure to HIV. Poverty and inequalities of several sorts are central to the risks people face (Farmer 1999; Loevinsohn and Gillespie 2003a).

Gender

Women are biologically, socioeconomically, and socioculturally more at risk of HIV infection than men. Gender inequity shapes power relations and sexual relations and thus risk. The subservient status of women is a central feature of the risk environments of southern and eastern Africa, and HIV/AIDS exacerbates these inequalities (UNAIDS 1999).

From a biological point of view, women are more susceptible to HIV infection than men. Evidence indicates that the pathogenesis of HIV-1 infection in women cannot be entirely inferred from what is known about HIV-1 infection in men. Women in Kenya were found, for example, to be infected with more genetically diverse viruses than men (Poss et al. 1995; Long et al. 2000). There is mounting evidence that the female genital tract can serve as a reservoir for HIV infection (Burger and Weiser 2001; Hart et al. 1999; Kovacs et al. 1999). Male-to-female transmission of HIV is two to four times more efficient than female-to-male (Mastro and de Vincenzi 1996; de Vincenzi 1994; Nicolosi et al. 1994). Hayes et al. (1995) calculated the cofactor effect of genital ulcer diseases to be approximately five times higher for male-to-female than for female-to-male transmission.

There is strong evidence that both ulcerative and nonulcerative sexually transmitted diseases (STDs) promote HIV transmission by augmenting HIV infectiousness and HIV susceptibility through a variety of biological mechanisms. These effects are reflected in the relative-risk estimates found in numerous prospective studies from four continents: these range from 2.0 to 23.5, with most clustering between 2 and 5 (Fleming and Wasserheit 1999; Rottingen et al. 2001; Galvin and Cohen 2004).

Women's relative powerlessness increases their risk of exposure. Women are less likely to negotiate condom use with husbands or other partners. Some men force girls to have sex in the mistaken belief that they can rid themselves of the virus. Practices such as genital mutilation and dry sex are highly risky for women. That the male partner is often considerably older than the female further increases the power differential. The norm of virginity and the culture of silence regarding sex restrict adolescent girls' access to information about sex and heighten the risk of sexual coercion (Collins and Rau 2000; Gupta et al. 2003).

Violence against women, especially forced or coerced sex, increases women's vulnerability to HIV/AIDS. In South Africa, Jewkes and Abrahams (2002) found that in the 17-to-48 age group there are 2,070 rape incidents per 100,000 women per year. Nonconsensual sex in marriage and dating relationships is believed to be very common but is usually not well reported in surveys. Forced sexual initiation is reported by almost a third of adolescent girls. In addition, coerced sex is a common problem in schools and workplaces and among peers. The threat of violence affects women's power and ability to negotiate the conditions of sexual intercourse, especially condom use. The threat of violence may also affect women's use of services such as testing for HIV and the extent to which they feel able to discuss their serological status with others and seek social support.

Women also have more limited access to health care and may receive inferior care. Studies of other infectious diseases show that women frequently wait longer than men before visiting health facilities. Recent research reveals the possibility that a similar pattern holds for HIV care (Mocroft et al. 2000; Prins et al. 1999).

Economically, women's dependence on men and their unequal access to resources, opportunities, and assets, including land, often place them at high risk. Relative economic disadvantage significantly increases the likelihood of a variety of unsafe sexual behaviors and experiences, according to findings from the 2001 report "Transitions to Adulthood in the Context of AIDS in South Africa," which surveyed 14- to 24-year-olds in KwaZulu Natal, South Africa (Hallman 2004). Low socioeconomic status not only increases the likelihood of a woman's exchanging sex for money or goods; it also raises female chances of experiencing coerced sex and male and female odds of having multiple sexual partners. In addition, it lowers female chances of abstinence, female and male age at sexual debut, condom use at last sex, and communication with most recent sexual partner about sensitive topics. Low socioeconomic status has more consistent negative effects on female than on male sexual behaviors; it also raises the risk of early pregnancy. Poorer young people, especially women, also have access to significantly fewer media sources for family planning information.

Transactional sex is increasingly being incorporated into *ganyu* (casual labor) contracts in Malawi. This tendency escalated during the 2002 food crisis, when the practice of *kusokola* (looking for food) became more common. Women are becoming more mobile and more at risk: Bryceson et al. (2004) report that some women routinely travel miles to grain mills to collect maize bran left after milling, and many also engage in transactional sex with men working at the mills. Demoralization from such a hand-to-mouth existence has led, in rural Malawi, to an increase in alcohol consumption that is also fueling the market for casual sex.

As well as being more *susceptible* to HIV, women are often more *vulnerable* to the postinfection impacts of AIDS. In central Malawi, Shah et al. (2001) found women in the patrilocal villages to be more vulnerable to food insecurity. A newly widowed woman is expected to leave her husband's village and has no control over land and other assets she may have been using jointly with her husband. The death of the husband thus often results in the dissolution and relocation of the household.

In some cultures "widow inheritance," whereby a woman is "inherited" by her deceased husband's brother, is the only way in which a woman can retain rights to her husband's land. This exposes her to a greater HIV risk. In Swaziland, widow inheritance and polygamy were among the more important social drivers of HIV spread (Whiteside et al. 2003). Nilses et al. (2000) in Zimbabwe and Boerma et al. (2003) in Kenya and Tanzania observed marital status to be an important risk factor, with divorced, widowed, or separated women having a higher risk of HIV infection. Upholding female property and inheritance rights can thus help prevent the spread of HIV. Promoting women's economic security and empowerment reduces their vulnerability to domestic violence, unsafe sex, and other AIDS-related risk factors (see Part 2).

Mobility

Mobility is a marker for enhanced risk. The movement of people itself is not inherently risky, but when single people move or families are split up—often as a consequence of poverty—the likelihood of their engaging in risky sexual practices tends to increase (Decosas and Adrien 1997; Barnett and Whiteside 1999; Whiteside et al. 2003; Hope 2001). Many of the points of intersection between households and services represent opportunities for the spread of infection. A recent study of HIV infection among women in urban South Africa showed that HIV prevalence was significantly higher among migrant women than nonmigrant women (Zuma et al. 2003). Cross-sectional comparative studies in Senegal and Guinea-Bissau (Lagarde et al. 2003), Tanzania and Zimbabwe (Boerma et al. 2003), and four cities in Kenya, Zambia, Benin, and Cameroon (Auvert et al. 2001) found mobility to be associated with risky behaviors and HIV prevalence. Bloom et al. (2002) in Tanzania and Shah et al. (2001) in Malawi have shown community mobility to be strongly associated with risk of HIV infection. In villages whose residents traveled a lot, spending several days a week outside the village, a higher proportion of households was affected by chronic illness. Most of these people relied on petty trade and vending outside their villages for a livelihood. At the national level, Stillwaggon (2000), in a cross-country regression analysis of Latin American and Caribbean countries, found urbanization and labor migration to be significantly correlated with HIV prevalence.

Orphanhood

Orphans are likely to be particularly susceptible to HIV. They are likely to be more food-insecure, more malnourished, and less healthy than nonorphans (Lundberg and Over 2000; Ainsworth and Semali 2000; Gilborn et al. 2001; Gertler et al. 2003; Deininger et al. 2001). Controlling for wealth and other factors, orphanhood also confers added risk for unsafe sexual behaviors (Hallman 2004).

"Men, money, and mobility" may have been among the most important drivers of the epidemic in its early days, but increasingly now poverty underpins the main risk factors. Bryceson et al. (2004) make an interesting observation on this: certain social groups in Malawi, despite knowing the risks, continued to engage in high-risk behaviors. They did so, the authors contend, to affirm their social identity and to deny that "anything they do makes a difference to what they perceive as a life of powerlessness and despair" (p. 17). The "culture of poverty," as documented by Oscar Lewis (1976) in Latin America, may thus be as significant as material poverty in motivating risky behaviors.

Malnutrition and HIV Transmission

The premise that high rates of HIV prevalence in Africa are mainly due to high levels of sexual activity has restricted policy interventions. Prevention of HIV is pursued predominantly through initiatives to change behavior, such as ABC ("Abstain, Be faithful, use a Condom").[2] Several studies stress the need to look beyond proximal factors of high-risk behavior in HIV transmission. Auvert et al. (2001), in a multicenter study, conclude that the differences in efficiency of HIV transmission, as mediated by biological factors, outweigh differences in sexual behavior in explaining the variation in rate of spread of HIV between four cities in Kenya, Zambia, Cameroon, and Benin. Stillwaggon (2002), in her pioneering work, found falling calorie and protein consumption and increasing inequality to be strongly correlated with HIV prevalence in 44 sub-Saharan African countries.

---

[2]The preceding discussion of the ubiquity of coerced sex also starkly exposes the limitations of ABC.

Malnutrition and HIV Transmission Efficiency in Adults

Nietszche's famous observation that "what doesn't kill us makes us stronger" is a fallacy with respect to malnutrition and its effects. Malnutrition weakens the immune system, increasing the risk of ill-health, which in turn can aggravate malnutrition. It is a vicious cycle (Scrimshaw et al. 1968; Tomkins and Watson 1989). Around half of all global preschool child deaths are attributable to the negative synergy of malnutrition and infectious disease, with a majority of deaths complicated by mild to moderate undernutrition (Pelletier et al. 1994). Both general (protein and energy) and micronutrient deficiencies are associated with significant defects in cell-mediated and humoral immunity, depressed cytokine production, lowered specific antibody production, and decreased phagocyte function (Tomkins and Watson 1989). Infections are thus longer-lasting and more severe in someone who is malnourished. They may also be more frequent.

Though few studies have investigated whether malnutrition increases the efficacy of horizontal disease transmission between adults, there is some suggestive evidence. In a 24-month nested case-control study of sexually active women in Rwanda, controlling for socioeconomic status, pregnancy, and genetic ulcer disease, weight loss in the first six months of the study was a significant predictor of eventual seroconversion (Moore et al. 1993). Malnutrition, particularly vitamin A deficiency, is also associated with an increased risk of STDs, including genital ulcers and cervical herpes simplex virus (HSV) shedding (Semba et al. 1998; Mostad et al. 2000), which in turn has been found to increase the risk of HIV transmission (World Bank 1993; Auvert et al. 2001). In contrast, in a study among HIV-negative Kenyan men, lower plasma vitamin A levels were associated with a decreased risk of HIV seroconversion (MacDonald et al. 2001). More research is clearly needed.

Maternal Nutritional Status and Vertical Mother-to-Child Transmission (MTCT) of HIV

Vertical transmission of HIV from mother to infant, which can occur during pregnancy, during delivery, or postnatally through breastfeeding, is a major factor in the continuing spread of HIV infection. Inadequate nutritional status may increase the risk of vertical HIV transmission by influencing maternal and child factors for transmission. Numerous studies have also reported that micronutrient deficiencies impair immune responses, weaken epithelial integrity, and are associated with accelerated HIV disease progression.

Many studies suggest that improved maternal micronutrient status may reduce vertical transmission of HIV by enhancing systemic immune function in the mother or fetus, reducing the rate of clinical, immunological, or viral progression in the mother, reducing viral load or the risk of viral shedding in genital secretions or breast milk, reducing the risk of low birth weight, or maintaining the integrity of the child's gastrointestinal tract. A number of studies that have examined these relationships are described here; others, which have looked at responses to interventions, are discussed later.

Maternal viral load and immune status. Maternal viral load, and consequently immune status (measured by CD4 cells/μL) of the mother are important predictors of in utero, intrapartum, and postnatal transmission of HIV (Leroy et al. 2001; John et al. 2001; Fawzi et al. 2002b). In a placebo-controlled study in West Africa, postnatal transmission was found to be 10 to 14 percent in mothers with baseline CD4 counts below 500 cells/μL but less than 3 percent among women with baseline CD4 counts of 500 cells/μL or more (Leroy et al. 2002). In a study in Tanzania, postnatal transmission risks were found to be 3.0 and 2.1 times greater in women with CD4 counts below 200 cells/μL and between 200 and 499 cells/μL, respectively, when compared with women who had CD4 counts of 500 cells/μL or more in pregnancy (Fawzi et al. 2002b). Many studies (both observational studies and placebo-controlled trials) suggest a positive relationship between intake of several nutrients, including vitamins B, E, and C (but not A), and CD4 counts (Fawzi et al. 1998; Coutsoudis et al. 1997; Semba et al. 1998).

Maternal placental and genital factors. Studies in rats suggest that poor nutritional status may impair placental integrity (Noback and Takahashi 1978) and promote transplacental transmission of HIV. Nutritional deficiency may result in weaker mucosal immunity and higher risk of viral load in the genital tract. Two studies in Kenya provide evidence that vitamin A deficiency among women increases the risk of HIV shedding in the lower genital tract (Mostad et al. 1997; John et al. 1997), thereby potentially increasing the risk of vertical transmission during delivery.

Maternal breast health. Subclinical and clinical mastitis are associated with a two- to fourfold increase in the risk of vertical transmission through breastfeeding as a result of increased viral shedding in breast milk (Semba and Neville 1999; Semba 2000). Nduati et al. (1995) in Kenya also show that the low plasma vitamin A concentrations of HIV-positive women during pregnancy are associated with a higher risk of viral shedding in breast milk.

Fetal/child gastrointestinal integrity, immunity, and prematurity. The integrity of the gastrointestinal mucosal lining of a fetus or child affects the risk of transmission of HIV through ingestion of infected amniotic fluid or infected breast milk and is also important for combating infections in general. Vitamin A and zinc deficiencies are associated with impaired barrier function of the gastrointestinal tract (GIT). Moreover, GIT integrity, as well as humoral and cellular components of mucosal immunity, is likely to be particularly compromised in preterm and low-birth-weight infants. Prematurity is associated with increased vertical transmission of HIV infection (Brocklehurst and French 1998; Landesman et al. 1996). Fawzi et al. in Tanzania (2001) found that babies who were HIV-negative at birth and born at or before 34 weeks of gestation were 2.2 times more likely to become infected during the intrapartum and early breastfeeding periods than those born at or after 37 weeks. In the same trial, Dreyfuss et al. (2001) observed maternal weight to be a significant predictor of birth weight and intrauterine growth retardation among HIV-positive women, signifying the importance of maternal nutrition in preventing poor birth outcomes and thus reducing MTCT risk.

Micronutrient status and MTCT. Observational studies in Malawi and Rwanda (Semba et al. 1994) suggest that low serum levels of vitamin A among HIV-infected pregnant women may be associated with a higher risk of vertical transmission of HIV. But out of the three studies in the United States, only one study (Greenberg et al. 1997) observed this relationship. These inconsistencies could be due to the limited ability of observational studies to tease out the causal effects of micronutrient status and disease progression. Low serum vitamin A levels may be a marker (not a cause) of an advanced stage of HIV disease and hence of transmission risk. Moreover, confounding of the results by different lengths of follow-up time or other predictors of transmission among vitamin-deficient and -sufficient groups could explain these findings.

Overall, one of the main factors determining the risk of mother-to-child transmission of HIV is the health and nutritional status of the mother. This is a finding with profound implications. We know that maternal immune status is strongly related to her nutritional status, which in turn is strongly associated with the birth weight and nutritional status of the infant (ACC/SCN 2000; Allen and Gillespie 2001). This is one fact that has not changed from pre-AIDS times: *better maternal nutrition clearly benefits both mother and child.*

Chapter 2

Impacts of HIV/AIDS on Food and Nutrition Security

Having examined the food- and nutrition-relevant determinants of the risk of individuals being exposed and infected with the virus, we now focus on the downstream effects of HIV/AIDS on food and nutrition security (the upper right quadrant of Figure 1). A plethora of studies on this topic have emerged in recent years. Many have employed a sustainable-livelihoods approach (see Figure 2), and many have found significant impacts on all the major classes of assets and capital, and on most institutions. Human capital is being eroded through the effects of premature illness and death on productive and reproductive labor and through the fracturing of intergenerational knowledge transfer. Social capital is being put under immense strain by HIV-related stigma and exclusion, increasing orphaning rates, and reduced incentives for collective action. Financial capital is being eroded as expenditures for health care and funerals increase and credit becomes harder to access. And physical and natural capital is being undermined as labor losses affect the ability to farm and maintain common property resources, and assets are sold off to raise cash.

Present knowledge of the more common impacts and responses relating to these five main asset classes at the household and community levels is summarized in Table 1. However, impacts vary significantly among different geographical areas and livelihood systems and with the degree of resilience demonstrated by households and communities.

In this section, we follow the logic in Figure 1 and trace the different waves of impacts of HIV/AIDS on food and nutrition security, from the micro to the macro levels.

Table 1 Commonly reported impacts of HIV/AIDS on livelihood and assets, and responses at household and community levels

Household level	Community level
Human impacts • Illness, malnourishment, and/or death of one or more household members • Change in size and composition of households; dependency ratio may increase • Children orphaned by the epidemic • Temporary migration for wage work • Loss of farm and off-farm labor • Reduced time available for domestic labor, including child care • Loss of agricultural knowledge, practices, and skills • Reduced quality and quantity of dietary intake (when nutrient requirements may be higher) • Increased malnutrition among adults and children (stunting, wasting)	• Increase in prevalence of illness • Loss of significant proportions of the population • Increased prevalence of child malnutrition • Shortage of experienced labor in all sectors of the economy • Increase in the price of labor • Increase in the number of female-, elderly-, and child-headed households • Increase in the number and rate of orphaned children • Change in outmigration of young adults • Change in age and sex composition • Reduction in school enrollment • Increase in school dropout rate • Loss of knowledgeable and experienced community leaders
Financial impacts • Reductions in income from farm and off-farm sources • Increased expenditure on health care, transport, and funerals • Reduced expenditure on agricultural inputs, e.g., fertilizer and seed • Liquidation of savings accounts; sale of livestock and assets, e.g., jewelry • Increased reliance on off-farm income • Reduced access to credit; increased debt • Borrowing from informal sector and/or from usurious money lenders; pledging of future crops	• Decrease in aggregate community income • Reduction in expenditures among community businesses • Reduction in aggregate community savings • Increase in demand for loans and consumption credit • Decrease in demand for productive credit • Increase in price of credit • Increase in default rate in credit markets • Increased spending on traditional and modern health care

Natural impacts	
• Reductions in soil fertility • Declines in on-farm conservation and/or irrigation practices • Fallow land returning to bush • Decline in quality of permanent crops • Renting or leasing out portions of land • Appropriation of land by relatives (taken from widows, orphans) • Sale of land and/or livestock	• Reduction in quality of community land resources • Decline in conservation of land and water resources • Decrease in biodiversity and genetic resources • Increase in fallow land • Change in land use, farming systems, and land markets • Environmental deterioration, e.g., reduced upkeep of terraces
Social impacts	
• Increased reliance on extended family and formal and informal community organizations for agricultural production, housework, child care, and fostering • Increased reliance on community willingness to support educational and nutritional needs of orphaned children (e.g., school fees, uniforms, and supplemental feeding) • Less time to participate in social and cultural activities • Possible disintegration of household	• Change and disruption of kinship and extended family ties, formal and informal organizations in the community, and labor-sharing arrangements • Increase in demand for community care for sick and dying members, apprenticeship training for orphaned adolescents, community social support, self-help organizations, child fostering, and child care • Increase in social inequality (e.g., through land acquisition) • Community fractionalization or disintegration (stigma)
Physical impacts	
• Decline in quality, or sale of, livestock, household goods, and tools, e.g., plows, housing	• Decline in condition of community infrastructure, such as wells, irrigation facilities, roads, drainage ditches, terraces, and schools

Sources: Gillespie et al. 2001; Stokes 2002; Harvey 2004.

Household Size and Composition

Households experiencing adult mortality tend to become permanently smaller than other households (Janjaroen 1998; Menon et al. 1998; Yamano and Jayne 2004), as some household members leave following an adult death. In Uganda, for example, household size fell by 1.7 members on average in households that experienced death, compared to a decline of 0.1 persons in other households (Menon et al. 1998).

Changes in household size and composition following a death are sensitive to the age, gender, and position of the deceased adult. In Kenya, when a female adult died, children were frequently sent to live with relatives, whereas the death of a male household head often led to daughters leaving the household on marriage (Yamano and Jayne 2004). Similarly, in a recent study in Mozambique, Mather et al. (2004a) found that after a female prime-age death, it is likely that children will leave the household and a new female adult will arrive.

Some households dissolve after a prime-age adult death. The death of a male head of household in Tanzania is more likely to cause dissolution of the household than the death of a female head (Urassa et al. 2001). Hosegood et al. (2003), in rural KwaZulu Natal, South Africa, found that 5 percent of 10,490 observed households experienced at least one AIDS-related death during the one-year observation period. These households were three times more likely to dissolve than other households. In Uganda, Ntozi (1997), in a retrospective study of the migration of spouses and other household members, found that 37 percent of widows and 17 percent of widowers migrated from their original homes (spousal death from AIDS-related causes ranged from about 50 to 60 percent). Younger spouses and those in worse health were more likely to leave. Women were more likely to leave because they were generally not entitled to inherit the land, and their kin often lived elsewhere. Even when it does not dissolve the household, death may cause dislocation of families: among the matrilineal people in rural Zambia, for example, women return with their children to their own mothers' villages (Drinkwater 1993).

In studies in Kenya and Mozambique, households were often unable or unwilling to replace their adult members after an adult death (Yamano and Jayne 2004; Mather et al. 2004a). In contrast, Rwandan households with an adult death were able to maintain their labor supply through addition of new members (Donovan et al. 2003). In Mozambique, households were more likely to hire or share labor after male deaths than after female deaths. Death of a household head increased the likelihood of the use of child labor.

One interesting finding of Michigan State University's comparative study of Kenya, Malawi, Mozambique, Rwanda, and Zambia was that, in four of the five countries, a majority of deceased prime-age adult deaths were *not* household heads or spouses (Mather et al. 2004b). This observation explains the low household dissolution rates in these studies. The authors suggest that the potential effect of prime-age mortality on agriculture may thus be less than is predicted by other studies, given that household heads and spouses tend to be the household members most heavily involved in agriculture. The demographic group most affected was younger female dependents.

The impact of mortality on household demographics may be much more severe when the adult death is due to HIV/AIDS than with other causes of death. Two person-years of labor may be lost because of the weakening of the person and the amount of time spent caring for him or her before death (FAO 2003a). Adverse dependency ratios were observed in households with the death of an HIV-positive adult but not with the death of an HIV-negative adult, and there was a significant association between child-headed households and adult death from AIDS (Menon et al. 1998). Floyd et al. (2003), in a retrospective cohort study in Malawi, investigated the effect of HIV on household structure over more than ten years. At the time of the follow-up survey, only one in five marriages in which one partner was HIV-positive at the outset was still intact. Children of HIV-positive parents were less likely to be alive and resident in the district than children of HIV-negative parents.

Child Survival and Nutrition

The impacts of HIV/AIDS on nutritional status can be viewed for different sub-sub-groups (adults and children) and at different levels (population and individual). Here we start with a population focus.

A recent study has shown that the 2002 drought in southern Africa interacted with HIV/AIDS in high-prevalence areas to bring about a rapid deterioration in child nutrition. Because this effect was observed mainly in areas that had previously had better child nutrition, the result was not so obvious when averages were viewed. Examining the situation in six countries—Lesotho, Malawi, Mozambique, Swaziland, Zambia, and Zimbabwe—Mason et al. (2003) found that HIV (more prevalent in urban areas) was leveling out the preexisting urban/rural nutritional differentials. They found some very large changes in child underweight prevalence, which increased from 5 percent to 20 percent in Maputo (Mozambique, 1997–2002), from 17 percent to 32 percent in Copperbelt (Zambia, 1999–2001/2), and from 11 percent to 26 percent in Midlands province (Zimbabwe, 1999–2002). Changes were much smaller during nondrought periods and in areas with lower HIV prevalences.

These trends may be due partly to the direct effects of pediatric AIDS (growth failure was seen at younger ages than previously), but the larger effect, the authors speculate, is probably indirect, with drought and HIV hastening destitution in affected families. Traditionally worse-off areas appeared protected, possibly in part because they received food assistance. The study points to the emergence of a vulnerable group in the better-off areas, to which resources need to be directed. Although the causes are yet to be determined, they may include poorer child care as well as food insecurity (for orphans and others) (Mason et al. 2003).

Maternal HIV status is also associated with mortality in young children—in Tanzania, for example, the mortality rate among children under two years of age born to HIV-positive mothers was 2.5 times higher than among children of HIV-negative mothers (Urassa et al. 2001). Adult mortality also adversely affects children's nutritional status. In Tanzania, children whose parents have died are more likely to be stunted (Lundberg and Over 2000; Ainsworth and Semali 2000). Children in the poorest households, those with uneducated parents, and those with the most limited access to health care are most severely affected. In Uganda, orphans' health and nutritional status were worse and their use of public services much lower than those of nonorphans (Deininger et al. 2003).

The type of orphanhood seems to matter. In Indonesia, maternal orphans had a 15 percent higher probability of being wasted than paternal orphans, and maternal (but not paternal) death also had a significant effect on child mortality. In Mexico, both paternal and maternal death were positively associated with child mortality (Gertler et al. 2003). In a study in Tanzania, Ainsworth and Semali (2000) show that the death of the mother was associated with an average decline of one standard deviation in child height-for-age between 1991 and 1994, whereas a paternal death was associated with a decline of one-third of a standard deviation. The impact of maternal orphanhood is severe regardless of household assets, while the impact on paternal orphans is felt only in poor households.

Individual Nutritional Status

Nutrition and immunity in HIV-positive individuals can interact in two ways. First, HIV-induced immune impairment and the heightened risk of subsequent infection can worsen nutritional status. HIV infection can also lead to nutritional deficiencies through decreased food intake and malabsorption and increased utilization and excretion of nutrients, which in turn hasten the onset of AIDS (Semba and Tang 1999). Nutritional status modulates the immunological response to HIV infection, affecting the overall clinical outcome. Teasing out the most important pathways is challenging because these relations are deeply intertwined, with many confounders (see Figure 3).

Immune suppression caused by protein-energy malnutrition is similar in many ways to the effects of HIV infection (Beisel 1996). Interestingly, the strong linkages between malnutrition and infection were decades ago referred to as nutritionally acquired immunodeficiency syndrome (Scrimshaw et al. 1968). AIDS itself during the 1980s was called "Slim," reflecting the characteristic wasting syndrome.

Figure 3 The vicious cycle of malnutrition and HIV

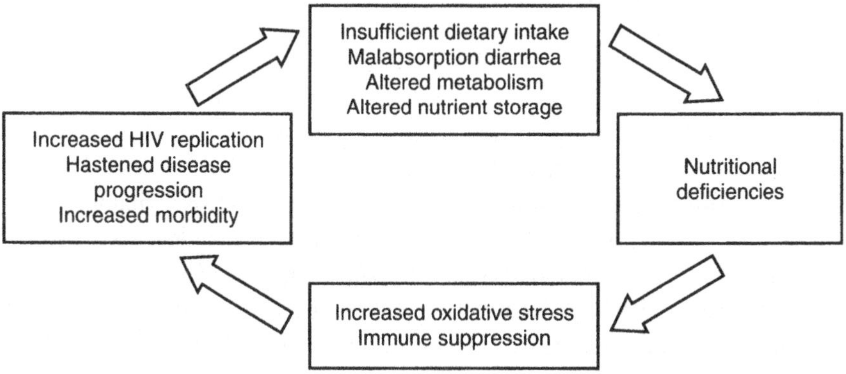

Source: Semba and Tang 1999.

General (protein-energy) malnutrition is associated with adverse clinical outcomes in people living with HIV in both the developed and the developing world. The relation between depletion of body cell mass and survival in adults with AIDS was first observed by Kotler et al. (1989), who hypothesized that the degree of malnutrition affected the clinical course and survival of these patients. Suttmann et al. (1995) showed that loss of body cell mass independently predicted death. In a U.S. study, Wheeler et al. (1998) found weight loss of 5 percent over a period of four months to be associated with an increased risk of death and opportunistic infections. In Malawi, a study of people with tuberculosis (80 percent of them HIV-positive) found that a body-mass index (BMI) of less than 17 increased the risk of early death (Zachariah et al. 2002). Losses in weight, fat-free mass, body cell mass, and fat mass were all significant predictors of mortality among HIV-positive persons with wasting syndrome in the Tufts Nutrition for Healthy Living Study in Boston (Tang 2003). Among HIV-positive Ugandan children, death before the age of 25 months was nearly five times more likely to occur among those with weight-for-age *z*-scores less than –1.5 than among those with higher *z*-scores (Berhane et al. 1997). There are thus convincing data showing a predictive link between malnutrition and adverse clinical outcomes, including death, in people living with HIV.

Micronutrient malnutrition, prevalent in many developing countries, may also contribute to a weakening of immune status and thus a worsening of clinical condition among HIV-infected individuals (Piwoz and Preble 2000; Fawzi 2003). There is substantial evidence that specific nutritional deficiencies may accelerate disease progression and hasten the onset of AIDS and death. Interactions between immune function and specific nutrient deficiencies in HIV-1 disease have been reported for trace elements (selenium and zinc) and vitamins A, E, B6, and B12.

Low levels of serum vitamin E and B12 were shown to prospectively increase disease progression (Tang et al. 1997a; Tang et al. 1997b; Baum 2000). Higher intakes of vitamin B (niacin, B1, B2, and B6) and vitamin C were associated with slower progression to AIDS (Tang et al. 1993; Tang et al. 1996). Selenium deficiency has been demonstrated to be a significant predictor of HIV-related mortality independent of CD4 cell count over time, CD4 cell count of less than 200 cells/μL at baseline, and antiretroviral treatment (Baum and Shor-Posner 1998).

No consistent relationship has been shown, however, between vitamin A and zinc deficiencies and HIV/AIDS. Vitamin A deficiency was an independent predictor of mortality among HIV-positive intravenous drug users (Semba et al. 1995). In a study among HIV-negative Kenyan men, lower plasma vitamin A levels were associated with a decreased risk of HIV seroconversion (MacDonald et al. 2001). In another prospective study among HIV-infected men in the United States, a U-shaped relationship was observed between dietary vitamin A intake and the risk of progression to AIDS and mortality (Tang et al. 1993; Tang et al. 1997a). These investigators also reported dietary zinc intake to increase the rate of disease progression and mortality. In contrast, those who progressed to AIDS in the study had significantly lower serum zinc levels than nonprogressors and HIV-negative subjects. More research is clearly needed.

Rural Livelihoods

Agriculture is the main source of livelihood for the majority of the people affected by HIV/AIDS around the world. In this section, we review the impacts of HIV/AIDS on subsistence and commercial agriculture and on agricultural extension capacity before turning to examine the impacts on off-farm livelihoods.

Subsistence Agriculture

The threat that HIV/AIDS poses for food security was first recognized in the late 1980s and early 1990s (Gillespie 1989; Barnett and Blaikie 1992; Brown et al. 1994). Many studies in sub-Saharan Africa, particularly over the last three to four years, show the vulnerability of subsistence agriculture to the impacts of AIDS. As Table 1 shows, these include reductions in the area of land under cultivation and crop diversity, abandonment of specific activities and crops, shifts to less labor-intensive monocultivation, use of minimum-tillage techniques, and reduced livestock use (e.g., FASAZ/FAO 2003; NAADS 2003; Drimie 2003). Below we summarize the main findings from different studies:

- In Rwanda, Donovan et al. (2003), in their descriptive analysis of a cross-sectional study with a four-year recall of household mortality information, found that 60 to 80 percent of rural-study households suffering illness or death reported reduced farm labor. (Household demographic information was collected only in 2002; household crop area and production information was collected in 2000, 2001, and 2002 for the same households.) Following a male death, households cultivated less land. In households with an ill or recently deceased adult male, cassava production rose 44 percent, and sweet-potato production increased 120 percent, but these crops declined if the female died. (Such tubers may have low labor intensity, but they are also low in nutritional value, with potential costs to health if they form the bulk of the diet over an extended period.) When a woman died or became ill, households were more likely to share or hire labor. About 50 percent reported their diets deteriorating.

- In a retrospective study from Kenya, Yamano and Jayne (2004), using a panel of 1,422 Kenyan households surveyed in 1997 and 2000, found the death of a prime-age male household head to be associated with a 68 percent reduction in per caput household crop production value. Adult female mortality caused a greater decline in cereal area cultivated, whereas prime-age male adult death resulted in a greater decline in cash crops (such as coffee, tea, and sugar) and nonfarm income. There is little indication that households recover quickly, though the authors observed that initial asset base does play a role in buffering the shock of adult mortality. Following the death of a male head, poor households reduced crop production, small livestock holdings, and nonfarm income. Nonpoor households suffered losses of nonfarm income only. Shah et al. (2001) made similar observations in Malawi.
- In Malawi, Shah et al. (2001) found 70 percent of the households affected by chronic sickness to be suffering from labor shortages, with 45 percent delaying agricultural operations and 25 percent leaving land fallow or changing the crop mix.
- In Zimbabwe, Kwaramba (1997) found output declines of 37 to 61 percent for different crops.
- In Swaziland, Muwanga (2002) found a reduction of 54 percent in maize production following the death of the household head.
- In Uganda, in an in-depth qualitative survey in three communities at different stages of HIV/AIDS impact and different farming systems, Barnett et al. (1995) found a progressive decline in production and socioeconomic status among affected communities.
- In a reconnaissance survey of 220 households, followed by an in-depth study of ten households with AIDS, Tibaijuka (1997) reported significant losses in agricultural production due to labor loss, and reallocation of labor to nurse the ill. Working capital was used to pay mounting medical bills.
- In Mozambique, a nationally representative survey with recall data on the

deaths, departures, and arrivals of household members between 1999 and 2002 found cash, livestock, assets, and total and per-adult-equivalent income to be lower for households experiencing death. Affected households had smaller total and cultivated land areas, particularly following the death of a male household head. But cultivated area per adult equivalent of the households experiencing death was similar to that of unaffected households because of net outmigration (Mather et al. 2004a).

- In Namibia and Uganda, widespread sale and slaughter of livestock to support the sick and to provide food for funeral mourners was found to have a detrimental effect on crop production (Engh et al. 2000; Haslwimmer 1994). After a male death, widows and children were left to take care of the livestock; they often lacked the management skills to do so effectively, further eroding this asset.

Among the key factors conditioning the nature and magnitude of impacts on agriculture are climate and rainfall patterns. In farming systems with only small windows of opportunity for undertaking essential, labor-intensive tasks such as planting or harvesting, farming households are particularly vulnerable, especially if surplus labor is not readily available. Using data from Rwanda, Gillespie (1989) projected AIDS mortality rates for different age and sex groups on the basis of epidemiological models and then related these to the different levels, type, and timing of typical farm labor for each group. He characterized the most vulnerable farming systems as those that exhibited a highly seasonal demand for labor, significant specialization of tasks by age and sex, a high interdependence of labor inputs, increasing returns to scale of labor, and limited ability to exchange labor for capital. Vulnerability relates strongly to the degree of substitutability of land, labor, and capital resources and flexibility in sequencing critical tasks.

Labor constraints may not be the major or the only constraints in many areas. HIV/AIDS is progressively decapitalizing affected communities (Jayne et al. 2003). The sale of assets and reduction of cash investment into agriculture is likely over time to narrow the strata of farmers producing surpluses and to increase socioeconomic inequality within communities. Gender inequality may also worsen as women increasingly curtail income-earning opportunities to care for those who are sick. Yamano and Jayne (2004) showed that on-farm labor gaps in rural Kenya were often filled by incoming household members, who therefore had to cease off-farm earning, potentially further exacerbating capital constraints.

Some rural studies have not found HIV/AIDS impacts on agriculture, though many of these were done over a decade ago, when the epidemic was in its relative infancy. In Kagera, Tanzania, Beegle (2003) showed that households experiencing adult mortality in the early 1990s did not suffer significant changes in labor supply.

They did not shift cultivation toward subsistence food farming and did not appear to have reduced the diversity of income sources more than six months after a death. This study did not, however, investigate whether these households were importing labor or whether food and nutrition outcomes were maintained. In another early 1990s study in Tanzania, Barnett et al. (1995) did not find any significant impact of AIDS on livelihoods. Those most affected were also most food-secure. Similarly, they found that in Zambia, the most affected households and communities were engaged in farming systems that were not particularly vulnerable to labor loss.

There is a dearth of studies on the impact of HIV/AIDS on livestock, fishing, pastoralism, and other livelihood systems. More research on this topic and on the interconnectedness of these sectors to subsistence agriculture is needed.

In sum, impacts of HIV/AIDS on agriculture differ by community and by household, in type and in degree. The nature and severity of impacts often depends on the age, gender, and position of the deceased in the household; whether lineage is matrilocal or patrilocal; the nature of the farming system and the degree of specialization it requires; and the overlap of HIV/AIDS and food security in that particular community.

Impacts are also dynamic: it would be interesting, for example, to see, as the epidemic has matured, whether food insecurity and HIV prevalence have converged in the Tanzania locale studied by Beegle (see above). Barnett and Topouzis (2003) differentiate three chronological stages in the epidemic—AIDS-initiating, AIDS-impending, and AIDS-impacted. In the early 1990s, many communities in eastern and southern Africa were still in the AIDS-impending phase, with many individuals infected but still asymptomatic. Ten years on, far more regions are AIDS-impacted, with widespread AIDS deaths and other consequences taking their toll.

Impacts may also be revealed in people's *responses* to the epidemic, and these too differ in effectiveness and sustainability. Some responses may be characterized as "coping," demonstrating resilience; others are clearly indicative of extreme duress and are not sustainable. This topic is discussed more fully later. One illustrative example of impact and responses is provided in Box 2.

Commercial Agriculture and the Private Sector

HIV/AIDS has profoundly impacted commercial agriculture (Rugalema 1999). In the studies cited below, illness and death were found to be the major reasons for employee exit from firms. The costs to employers include replacement worker costs, paid sick leave, lost wages, and productivity losses. In Kenya, the medical expenditures incurred by agricultural companies due to HIV/AIDS increased by US$1.15 million between 1989 and 1995 (Rugalema 1999). Guinness et al. (2003) in Zambia confirm the high costs that employers and employees incur as a result of HIV/AIDS.

Box 2. Dynamics of HIV/AIDS impacts and household responses in an agriculture-based livelihood

The following is an illustration of *possible* impacts and responses of an agriculture-dependent household containing an adult who contracts HIV. Context will obviously influence the type and sequence of events and responses.

- Adult becomes sick
- S/he reduces work
- Replacement labor is "imported," perhaps from relatives
- Adults work longer hours on farm
- Health-care expenses rise (e.g., drugs, transport)
- Household consumes less food
- Farming switches to less labor-intensive crops and farming systems, small livestock
- Nutritional status deteriorates
- Adult stops work
- Household devotes more care to sick adult, less to children
- Small assets are disposed of (e.g., livestock)
- Debts increase
- Children drop out of school to help with household labor
- Adult dies
- Funeral expenses are incurred
- Household fragments as other adults migrate for work
- Household reduces cultivation of land, leaves more fallow
- Inappropriate natural-resource management leads to spread of pests and disease
- Effects of knowledge loss intensify
- Common property resources are mined
- Surviving family members lose access to land and property (e.g., surviving widow)
- Solidarity networks become strained, possibly to point of exclusion
- Partner becomes sick
- Downward spiral accelerates

Source: Gillespie et al. 2001.

And in a study of male sugar-mill workers in South Africa, Morris et al. (2000) project a tenfold increase in costs due to HIV/AIDS for companies between 2000 and 2006.

But, as Rosen and Simon (2002) highlight, "burden-shifting" is becoming more common. The private sector can avoid the economic burden of AIDS more readily than governments, households, or nongovernmental organizations (NGOs) and has systematically set about doing so. Shifting the AIDS burden from businesses to households and government is accomplished by such practices as preemployment health screening, reducing employee benefits, restructuring employment contracts, outsourcing less skilled jobs, selective retrenchments, and making changes in production technologies. In South Africa, more than two-thirds of large employers have reduced health-care benefits or required larger employee contributions. Most firms have replaced defined-benefit retirement funds, which expose the firm to large annual costs but provide long-term support for families, with defined-contribution funds, which eliminate risk to the firm but provide little to families of younger workers who die of AIDS (Rosen and Simon 2002).

A recent study of tea-estate workers in Kenya is one of the first to rigorously quantify the impact of HIV/AIDS on individual labor productivity (Fox et al. 2004). A retrospective cohort design was employed to study the productivity and attendance of tea-estate workers who died or retired because of AIDS-related causes between 1997 and 2002 in western Kenya. After adjusting for age and environmental factors, results showed that HIV-positive individuals plucked 4 to 8 kg/day less in the last 18 months before termination. They used significantly more leave days and spent more days doing less strenuous tasks in the two years before termination than did other pluckers. Those who stopped working because of AIDS-related causes earned 16 percent less in their second year before termination and 18 percent less in the year before termination. These results show that the drop-off is significant and starts years before the employee has to terminate work. They may, in fact, underestimate productivity losses, as workers often bring unrecorded "helpers."

Agricultural Extension

HIV/AIDS is also significantly impacting agricultural extension services. HIV prevalence rates among ministry of agriculture (MoA) staff are likely to be at least as high as national average estimates, and most likely higher. In Kenya's MoA, 58 percent of all deaths in the late 1990s were thought to have been AIDS-related (GTZ 1999). In Malawi in 1998, at least 16 percent of the staff of the Ministry of Agriculture and Irrigation (MoAI) were reported to be living with HIV/AIDS, 76 percent had lost at least one colleague, and 60 percent had lost at least one close relative to AIDS (Bota et al. 1998, cited in Topouzis 2003). In Zambia, 67 percent (of 155) agricultural extension workers interviewed had lost at least one coworker to HIV/AIDS in the three years preceding one study (Alleyne et al. 2001).

Studies have also reported reductions in agricultural extension service time due to HIV/AIDS. Engh et al. reported a 10 percent decline in livestock extension service time in Namibia, and Haslwimmer (1994) in Uganda reported 25 to 50 percent reductions in agriculture extension time. In the mid-1990s, Haslwimmer (1994) found that up to half of agricultural extension staff time in one district in Uganda had been lost to HIV/AIDS. Staff members were frequently absent from work because they had to care for sick relatives or attend funerals, or were sick themselves.

Organizations in areas with a high HIV/AIDS prevalence are characterized by high absenteeism, high turnover, a loss of institutional memory, and reduced innovation. As individuals in government and NGOs continue to die, the capacity gap—between what is needed and what can be delivered—is becoming an abyss.

Nonagricultural Livelihoods

Most African households derive some income from nonagricultural activities (Reardon 1997; Bryceson 1999; Barrett and Reardon 2000; Ellis 2000). Surveys conducted during the 1980s and early 1990s estimated that roughly 40 percent of African rural household income was derived from nonfarm sources (Reardon 1997; Ellis 1998). By contrast, the 1995–97 DARE (De-Agrarianisation and Rural Employment) study of the University of Leiden, which studied households in Nigeria, Ethiopia, Tanzania, Congo-Brazzaville, Malawi, Zimbabwe, and South Africa, found that much higher levels (55 to 80 percent) of income were derived from nonfarm sources (Bryceson 2000). Surveyed households in the seven countries, on average, pursued two or more nonagricultural activities simultaneously. The role of the male head of household as the primary income-earner was found to be eroding. Rural women are increasingly earning cash from sales of prepared snacks, beer, hair plaiting, petty retailing, knitting, tailoring, soap making, midwifery, and prostitution. In Nigeria, data showed an increase in nonfarm activities from 33 percent of surveyed households in the mid-1980s to 57 percent in 1997. Among the poorest income group, participation increased from 37 percent to 80 percent; in the wealthiest income group, it decreased from 33 to 25 percent.

Much attention has been paid to the role of nonfarm livelihoods in coping with natural and policy shocks (Reardon et al. 1992; Ellis 1998), though little is known about the links between HIV/AIDS and such livelihoods. Studies reviewed earlier show that livelihoods involving migration or mobility increase the probability of risky behaviors. In terms of the impacts of AIDS, a reduction in prime-age adults in the household may permanently reduce off-farm income, as other family members are less likely to replace adults earning money at other sites. Yamano and Jayne (2004) found significant reduction in off-farm income following the death of male household heads in poor families. In Mozambique, Mather et al. (2004a) found significant reductions in off-farm income after the death of a male household head and also after the death of a female non-head adult. In Zambia and Malawi, households with the death of a non-head had lower mean incomes than those with the death of a head (Mather et al. 2004b).

There have been several impact studies that focus on outcomes relevant to food and nutrition but are not specific to agriculture. These tend to show that households with adult mortality are generally poorer, have lower food expenditures and higher medical bills, consume less food than other households, and are less likely to have their children in school.

Income

In a cross-sectional comparison of households with and without an HIV-positive individual in Free State, South Africa, per caput income in AIDS-afflicted households was 50 to 60 percent that of unafflicted households (Booysen and Bachmann 2002). In another cross-sectional survey of 680 households in Limpopo province, Oni et al. (2002) made similar observations. In a five-year retrospective study of 232 urban and 101 rural AIDS-affected families, Nampanya-Serpell (2000) reported a decline in monthly disposable income of more than 80 percent in more than two-thirds of the AIDS-affected families, with higher losses following a paternal death. But Urassa et al. (1997) found that in Tanzania, households with orphans did not have a lower economic status than those without orphans (though this may be a positive selection bias, as households with greater resources are more likely to foster orphans).

Household Consumption and Expenditure

Reducing food consumption quantity or quality may be a highly erosive "coping" strategy, as nutrient requirements rise following HIV infection (see below). In a panel study in Indonesia, Gertler et al. (2003) showed a prime-age male death to be associated with a 27 percent reduction in mean per caput household consumption, whereas the death of a female had no significant impact. In Mexico, they found the death of a prime-age adult household member to reduce per caput consumption by nearly 8 percent, with no significant gender differences.

In Côte d'Ivoire, Bechu (1998) surveyed 107 households with at least one adult ill with AIDS and with one or more children and interviewed them six times at two-month intervals. These data were compared with the results of a study conducted in Yopougon in May 1992 and based on a sample of 2,064 households. The study found per caput consumption of AIDS-afflicted households to be half that of other households. And in a cross-sectional survey of 119 households in the Rungwe district of Tanzania, Mwakalobo (2003) found that households that experienced an

AIDS death spent substantially less on food than other households. HIV/AIDS-related death significantly increased the probability of a household falling below the poverty line.

In South Africa, average monthly per caput food expenditure of afflicted households was 70 to 80 percent that of other households (Booysen and Bachmann 2002), but no significant difference was found in total monthly expenditures, most likely because of rises in health-related expenditures.

AIDS-afflicted households do tend to incur high health-care expenditures (Tibaijuka 1997 in Tanzania; Booysen and Bachmann 2002 in South Africa). Bechu (1998) in Côte d'Ivoire found that health-care costs specific to the person with AIDS accounted for almost 80 percent of the household health-care budget. In the Rungwe district of Tanzania, rising medical expenses or an HIV/AIDS-related death significantly increased the probability of a household's falling below the poverty line (Mwakalobo 2003).

Many studies show that households experiencing adult death tend not to recover to preshock levels of consumption (e.g., Yamano and Jayne 2004; Gertler et al. 2003; Bechu 1998). Such a lack of resilience is likely to increase vulnerability to other shocks to food and nutrition security (see "HIV/AIDS and Food Crises" below).

Education

Many studies have reported the negative effects of HIV/AIDS on children's schooling (Urassa et al. 1997; Gilborn et al. 2001; Yamano and Jayne forthcoming; Deininger et al. 2003; Gertler et al. 2003). Deininger et al. (2003), in an analysis of a panel data set of 1,300 households included in surveys conducted in 1992 and 2000, show that foster children were at a distinct disadvantage in both primary- and secondary-school attendance before the introduction of universal primary education. In Uganda, in a descriptive analysis of a baseline survey of 353 HIV-positive parents, 495 children of people living with HIV/AIDS (PLWHAs), 233 orphans, and 326 guardians, Gilborn et al. (2001) found declining school attendance among 28 percent of the older children of PLWHAs, whereas it was improving for 21 percent of older foster children.

In a recent study, Case et al. (2004) using 19 Demographic and Health Surveys (DHS) conducted between 1992 and 2000, examine the effect of orphanhood on children's school enrollment in 10 sub-Saharan African countries. Although poorer children are less likely to attend school, poverty alone does not account for the lower enrollment of orphans: orphans are less likely to be enrolled than are nonorphans with whom they live. Outcomes for orphans depend on the closeness of kin bonds to their household heads. The lower enrollment of orphans is largely explained by the greater tendency of orphans to live with distant relatives or unrelated caregivers.

Gertler et al. (2003) found that orphans are less likely to start school and more likely to drop out. Yamano and Jayne (forthcoming) found the negative impact of adult mortality on school attendance in Kenya to be more severe in poor households, as did Nampanya-Serpell (2000) in urban but not in rural areas of Zambia.

Yamano and Jayne (forthcoming) also found adult mortality negatively affecting schooling even in the period directly before the death, most likely because children are sharing the burden of caregiving.

Again, the type of orphanhood seems to matter. In Indonesia only maternal death resulted in delayed school entry, whereas paternal death increased the dropout rate; exactly the reverse occurred in both cases in Mexico (Gertler et al. 2003).

HIV/AIDS and Food Crises

The 2001–3 southern African food crisis generated the following two questions:

- How does HIV/AIDS contribute to food crises?
- What does this imply for the type of responses that are required?

The immediate triggers of the crisis were climatic. Flooding and poorly distributed rainfall in the first half of 2001 led to a reduction in food production across the five most severely affected countries. Multiple, overlapping factors exacerbated these impacts: deep and widespread poverty, civil strife and insecurity about land (in Zimbabwe), removal of price controls, resource degradation, erosion of agricultural diversity, poor governance, and repression of the press and civil society (Loevinsohn and Gillespie 2003b).

One factor that was more significant in this crisis than in past crises (e.g., the one in 1992) was HIV/AIDS. The region affected by the 2001–3 crisis has the highest rates of HIV infection in the world, and among the highest rates of poverty and malnutrition (see Loevinsohn and Gillespie 2003b; Table 2).

It is simplistic to ask whether AIDS causes famine. AIDS and other contributory factors are embedded in social, economic, and cultural systems and processes to an extent that makes relative attribution impossible. Multiple, negative synergies are at play. Yet there is growing recognition that the spread of HIV/AIDS has increased the sensitivity of agrarian society to the point where small shocks can precipitate crises for many people.

De Waal and Whiteside (2003) have posited a "new-variant famine" hypothesis in which hunger and HIV/AIDS reinforce each other with catastrophic consequences (see Box 3).

Figure 4 depicts this relationship in another way, plotting HIV prevalence against acute food insecurity. The new-variant hypothesis would suggest that

Table 2 Characteristics of countries in southern Africa hit by food shortages

	Percent adults living with HIV	Percent living in poverty[a]	Percent children underweight[b] (year of survey)	Percent (millions) of population in need of food aid, mid-2003
Malawi	15	85	25.4 (2000)	29 (3.2)
Zambia	21	87	25.0 (1999)	26 (2.9)
Zimbabwe	35	64	13.0 (1999)	49 (6.7)
Lesotho	31	66	17.9 (2000)	30 (0.65)
Swaziland	33	—	10.3 (2000)	24 (0.26)

[a]Defined as living on less than US$2 per day.

[b]Defined as weight for age < –2 *z*-score.

Sources: HIV: UNAIDS (http://www.unaids.org/hivaidsinfo), 2003. Food aid: WFP assessment briefs (http://www.wfp.org/newsroom/in_depth/Africa/southern_africa020705.htm). Poverty: World Bank 2002, Table 2.6. Nutrition: UNICEF (http://www.childinfo.org/eddb/nutrition.htm and http://childinfo.org/MICS2/natlMICSrepz/MICSnatrep.htm).

high HIV prevalence without acute food insecurity (top left) might undermine vulnerability over time, whereas acute food insecurity without high HIV prevalence (bottom right) might still be managed with traditional coping strategies. The new-variant famine might be expected to materialize where high HIV prevalence and acute food insecurity coexist (top right). The figure also shows how this dangerous coexistence may be reached through two routes, which themselves may become increasingly intertwined: increasing HIV spread in a situation of acute food insecurity, and increasing food insecurity where HIV prevalence is high.

If new-variant famines are hypothesized as being qualitatively and quantitatively quite different from "normal" famines, they demand qualitatively and quantitatively different responses.

Here it is worth taking a look at current disaster theory. Wisner et al. (2004) convincingly argue that disasters should not be regarded as separate from everyday living. Because the risks involved in disasters are connected with "normal" vulnerabilities, they are as much the product of social, political, and economic environments as of natural events per se. According to the pressure-and-release model (PAR), a disaster occurs at the intersection of two opposing forces: processes generating vulnerability on one side and the natural-hazard event on the other. The risk of disaster is a compound function of the severity of the natural hazard and the number of people vulnerable, in varying degrees, to that specific hazard:

Risk = *Hazard* × *Vulnerability*

The "pressure" is thus exerted from both sides, as with a nutcracker. "Release" may come through a reduction of vulnerabilities, which relieves the pressure. As

Box 3. HIV/AIDS and famine

Unlike "normal" or pre-AIDS famines, an "AIDS-affected famine" or new-variant famine (De Waal and Whiteside 2003) is likely to radically alter household dependency ratios. "Normal" famines kill the weakest first, that is, young children and the elderly, who are usually dependents. Households and communities are much better adapted for survival when the dependency ratio does not rise much or even falls. Coping—which hinges at some point on available labor—is possible.

An AIDS-affected famine is different because it will also kill the strong and the able-bodied. People who were infected before the onset of the food crisis will die more quickly if drought exacerbates their already worsening nutritional status. As a result, the dependency ratio may rise significantly. If sick and dying adults are also (and appropriately) counted as dependents, the ratio will be even higher: the notion of effective dependency ratio better accommodates this reality. This difference will have particularly severe consequences for women, who have greater total (domestic and external) work burdens than men, yet are more likely than men to become infected with HIV (more susceptible) and more likely to die sooner (more vulnerable).

The dependency ratio is further worsened by another AIDS-related trend: the common tendency for HIV-positive adults, cast off by the urban sector (public and private) because of their HIV status, to return to die in their villages. This trend places a "double burden of care" on rural households.

By Sen's reasoning, such heightened HIV-affected dependency ratios alone will increase the risk of collapse of a household's entitlement set (both endowments and exchange entitlement) (Sen 1981). A high prevalence of HIV/AIDS therefore is likely to significantly increase both the upstream susceptibility and the downstream vulnerability to famine.

Resilience (the ability to bounce back or recover) is likely to be seriously affected. A common early coping strategy is to fall back on the family network, but in high-HIV areas this may already be under extreme pressure. The next fallback is to labor power—again, not a viable option for AIDS-afflicted households. Even the gathering of wild foods requires knowledge gained over the years and passed down from parents to children—lifesaving knowledge that will now die with the parents. Reducing food consumption is not likely to be a survival strategy for many AIDS-afflicted households; it is more likely to hasten death. One of the last resorts, often irreversible, is to sell major assets, such as land or livestock, a step that seriously increases the risk of destitution and even starvation. And, finally, one of the most insidious aspects of the HIV/AIDS pandemic is that the last option left for a woman may be to trade sex for cash to feed her children. Severe vulnerability here has led to extreme susceptibility.

Wisner et al. point out, the new-variant famine hypothesis is compatible with the PAR model (2004, p. 189). But what is distinctive about HIV/AIDS in this context is that it may exert an influence on *both* sides of the nutcracker: that is, as prevalences increase, the biological hazard worsens, and as AIDS impacts grow, vulnerabilities increase. Another salient factor is the length of exposure to this hazard. As Wisner et al. observe, HIV/AIDS is a slow-onset disaster, and we have spoken of its long-wave nature. Unlike a flood, this particular hazard will be around for a long time.

Figure 4 AIDS, food crises, and famine

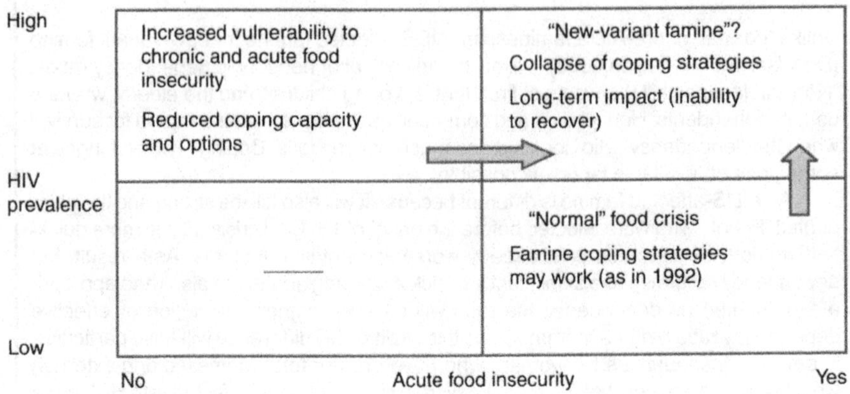

But what does the evidence show? Analyzing data from emergency food-security assessments conducted in Malawi and Zambia (in August and December 2002) and Zimbabwe (in August 2002), a recent study suggests that the impacts of HIV/AIDS on food security during the 2002 food emergency were strong, negative, and complex, demanding a rethinking of future responses (SADC FANR 2003). Households affected by adult morbidity and mortality and with a high demographic load were significantly more vulnerable to food-security shocks than other households were. They suffered from marked reductions in agricultural production and income, leading to earlier engagement in distress coping strategies, and, ultimately, a decline in food security. AIDS-affected households will take longer to recover from food crises and in fact may never recover completely. The analysis further demonstrates that different morbidity, mortality, and demographic profiles have different effects on food-security processes and outcomes, with implications for early warning systems.

In contrast, another study in Zambia found that HIV/AIDS had no impact on food production, although AIDS-affected households were more likely to cite lack of labor as a reason for limiting land cultivation than were unaffected households. Responses included changes in food consumption (Zambia VAC and SADC FANR 2003). In another Zambian assessment, Scott and Harland (2003) concluded that the food deficit was overestimated and the capacity of Zambian households to cope underestimated.

Although we do not know whether, when, or where "new-variant famine" scenarios will play out, they remain entirely plausible. But such crises do not develop out of the blue. Rather, they derive from a progressive intensification of long-term processes that compound the vulnerabilities of households and communities. These processes are fueled by many factors, now including HIV/AIDS. The dichotomy between development and humanitarian programming is a false one in the context of HIV/AIDS. The United Nations has spoken of the need for "emergency development" or "developmental relief" in this context (United Nations 2004).

Case Study: HIV/AIDS in India

Before we review possible responses to these interactions in Part 2, we examine the emerging situation in the Indian subcontinent, drawing on recent work by Kadiyala and Barnett (2004).

AIDS festers on the fault lines of societies, throwing into sharp relief inequalities between rich and poor, urban and rural, educated and uneducated, and men and women (Barnett and Whiteside 2002). As India shares the inequalities that drive the spread of the epidemic elsewhere in the world, it is not surprising that approximately 5.1 million people in India are living with HIV/AIDS, a total second only to that of South Africa (UNAIDS/UNICEF/WHO 2004; NACO 2004).

With India's deepening involvement in the globalized economy, and markets reaching into ever more remote parts of the country, the pressures to migrate, the opportunities to seek work, and the social and economic niches in which the virus may lodge will continue to increase. Many of the factors that increase the risk of HIV exposure are present in India: marked socioeconomic and gender inequalities, a high degree of population mobility, and high levels of poverty. Forty-four percent of the Indian population live below the international poverty line, and India ranks 127th out of the 175 countries in the Human Development Index (HDI).

India is also urbanizing rapidly, with nearly one-third of the population now living in urban areas (UNDP 2003). Most of these are migrant workers with families in rural areas. A study of migrant workers in Mumbai (where 46 percent of workers are migrants) and Delhi (where 65 percent are migrants) found that men not living with family were twice as likely to report visiting commercial sex workers as those living with families. The virus thrives in an environment of highly transient urban dwellers (Hira et al. 1998; Bhattacharjee et al. 2000).

The inferior material and cultural position of Indian women is indicated by the highly masculinized sex ratio and higher rates of illiteracy and child undernutrition among females. Because women have more limited access to economic opportunities, they are less likely to leave a relationship they perceive as risky. Indian norms of masculinity condone experimentation, extramarital affairs, and men's sexual domination over women; these practices increase men's risk of HIV as well as that of their partners. A large proportion of Indian women in monogamous marriages are increasingly susceptible to HIV (Hawkes and Santhya 2002; Newman et al. 2000).

Most research on susceptibility in India is based on a public-health model and relates to clinical and medical issues of prevention, access, and treatment. A few studies report on the practices of population subgroups, such as sex workers, students, teachers, and nurses (Ambati et al. 1997; Agarwal et al. 1999; Bhattacharjee et al. 2000; Lal et al. 2000; Thomas et al. 2002).

Only a handful of studies in India examine the socioeconomic well-being of households affected by HIV/AIDS (Basu et al. 1997; Gupta 1998; Bharat and Aggleton 1999). They show that affected households face severe constraints, mainly because of reduced income and increased health expenditures. Bloom and Mahal (1996) and Bloom and Glied (1993) examined the annual treatment costs of HIV/AIDS for households in nine Asian countries in the mid-1990s and concluded that, in most cases, these costs were more than twice the per capita income in each country (and these estimates exclude the costs of antiretroviral drugs). Bloom and Mahal (1997) predict that economic costs of AIDS will be felt not by nations but rather by households. Basu et al. (1997) report that health expenditure by households is four to five times higher than the state expenditure. They also report reduced consumption of milk, meat, and eggs as a result of increased health-care expenditures. Gupta (1998) shows that 10 to 30 percent of the annual income of an individual may be spent on the treatment of illness.

These few studies were conducted in urban areas, and we still know little about the epidemic in the rural areas. To respond with effective mitigation strategies, we need to know more about household response mechanisms in diverse settings. For example, how do Indian households deal with adult deaths? What are the implications of adult sickness and death for children in the household? What are the nature and magnitude of the gender differential of the epidemic? What are the implications of HIV/AIDS for social cohesion? How will orphans be supported?

It is expected that household-level impacts will translate to sectoral-level impacts. Studies on the sectoral impacts of HIV/AIDS are sparse, and the few that exist are mostly limited to the transportation industry. They show HIV/AIDS as having significant effects on the trucking industry even in the early stages of the epidemic (see, for example, Kanjilal 1995). The private sector has tended to adopt a wait-and-see attitude, with little intervention to anticipate and stem the spread and effects of the epidemic among employees (Bharat et al. 2001). More recently, multinational companies in India and a few large Indian corporations have started instituting HIV/AIDS-related workplace policies. Considering that the most susceptible and vulnerable population works in the small-scale, informal, and unorganized sectors, much more remains to be done.

These household- and sectoral-level impacts translate to macro effects on the economy that affect GDP growth rate. Studies indicate that increased medical costs represent high costs to the economy. Lost labor productivity could be as much as 1 percent of GDP (Pandav et al. 1997; Anand et al. 1999). But these estimates only refer to the costs accounted for in formal economics. There are far more diverse and greater costs, borne by individuals and households, that are not counted (Barnett 2004).

Part 2

Responses

We now move from mapping the interactions to looking at what can be done, and what is actually being done, to address them. Part 2 comprises four sections:

1. a process for moving from understanding interactions to responding to them;
2. examples of such responses, ranging from community responses to appropriate policy modifications and new interventions;
3. a discussion of the challenges of mainstreaming, scaling up, and capacity development; and
4. a consideration of next steps and conclusions.

Chapter 3

Applying an HIV/AIDS Lens

One tool to help move from understanding to responding is the HIV/AIDS lens, developed by Loevinsohn and Gillespie (2003a) in the context of the emerging RENEWAL initiative (www.ifpri.org/renewal).[3] This approach incorporates the concepts described above, the generic map in Figure 1, and the current state of knowledge of the interactions between food and nutrition security and HIV/AIDS in any given situation. The lens is designed to support reflection on how a particular situation or particular policy may be increasing or reducing the risks people face either of contracting HIV or of suffering severe consequences from AIDS-linked illness and death. It thus helps clarify options for response.

The lens is bifocal in the sense that it focuses on both the upstream factors of susceptibility and resistance and the downstream factors of vulnerability and resilience (see Figure 5, which is essentially a simplification of Figure 1). It may be used internally, within the workplace, or externally, on policies and programs. It can help reveal trade-offs as well as positive-sum solutions, and it is both context-specific and dynamic: it can evolve over time, as our knowledge of these interactions develops.

A process for using the lens to re-view food and nutrition policies is illustrated in Figure 6. First, HIV/AIDS and food and nutrition security are analyzed to summarize what is known about the nature and extent of their interactions and what forms of institutional response currently exist. This analysis helps construct the lens. Second, key policies and programs are reviewed in terms of their potential contribution—positive or negative—to HIV/AIDS prevention and mitigation. This review may be carried out in workshops, by the researchers, program managers, or

[3]Much of this section derives from Loevinsohn and Gillespie 2003a.

Figure 5 A bifocal lens

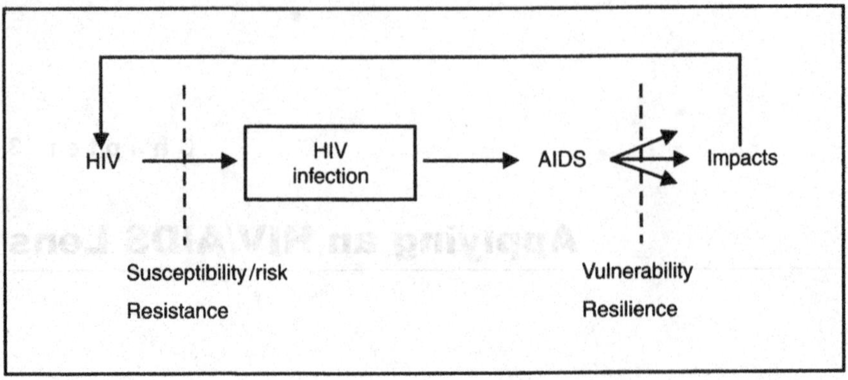

policymakers responsible for them, with outside facilitation and the involvement of key stakeholders. Participants ask questions that focus on two issues:

Prevention. How might this policy or program be increasing people's susceptibility (or resistance) to HIV infection?

Mitigation. How might this policy or program be increasing people's vulnerability (or resilience) to the impacts of AIDS?

The result of this review will be a list of policies and programs prioritized according to their potential positive or negative contribution to HIV/AIDS prevention and mitigation. Depending on the state of existing knowledge, further field-level evidence may be required prior to policy modification, or enough may be known to take action. Action research in the field involves gathering quantitative and qualitative evidence on whether the policy or program is helping or hindering affected households in avoiding HIV risks and dealing with AIDS impacts. Subsequently the policy or program may be modified, drawing on the results of these field assessments, with changes made across a spectrum ranging from changing nothing to changing everything (that is, stopping the existing program and initiating a new one). Different aspects of a program—the what, how, who, and where—may need to change. In some cases, the changes can be made at full scale, whereas others may have to be tested with pilot programs. Whatever changes are made, it is critically important to monitor the effects of the revised policies and use the results to refine the lens.

The lens is flexible and adaptive: it may be used in different ways by a range of actors, not just policymakers. At the community level, the lens can also be used to reveal options for relevant responses.

Figure 6 Using an HIV/AIDS lens to improve policy

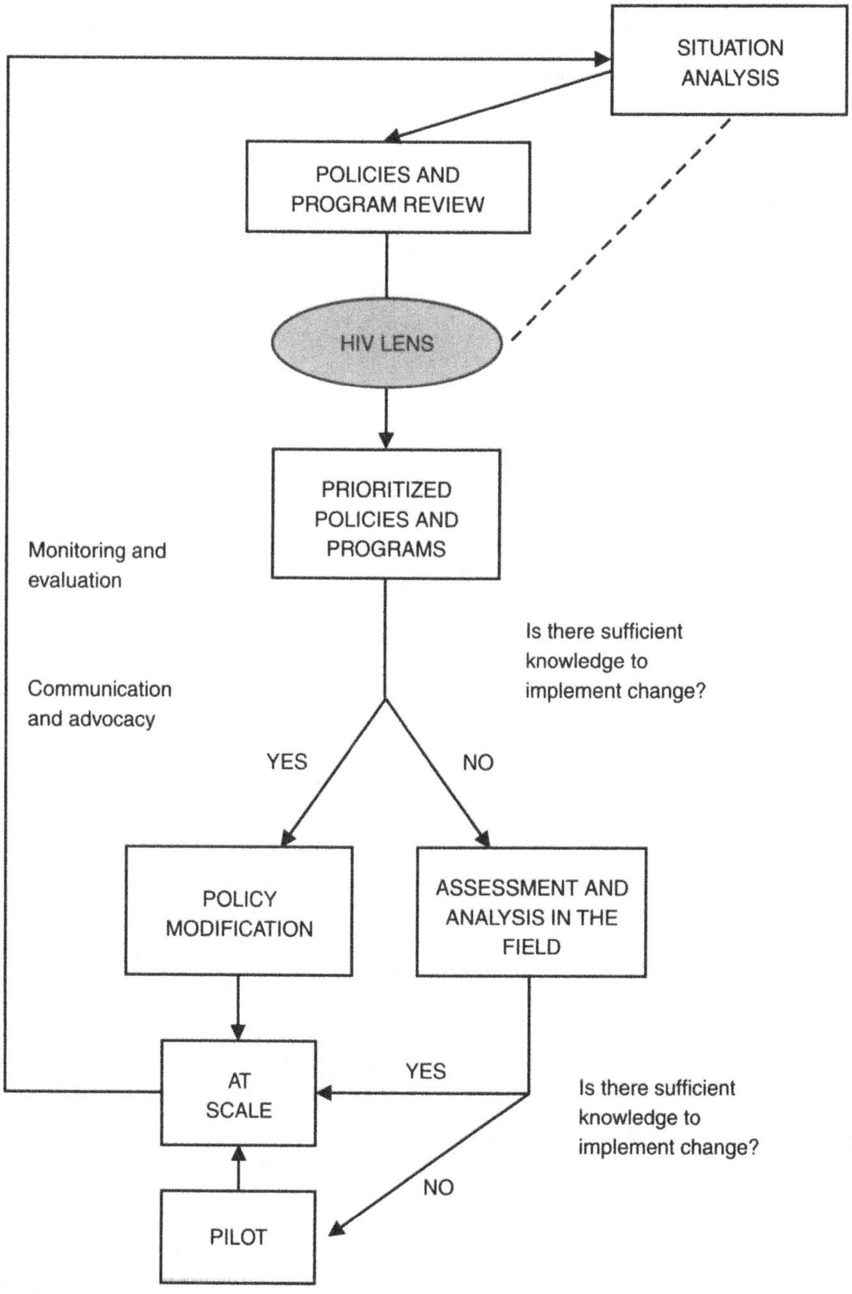

Source: Loevinsohn and Gillespie 2003a.

Given the interactions between food and nutrition insecurity and HIV/AIDS, it will also be important for a food and nutrition lens to be applied to HIV-specific programming. We discuss this approach in the contexts of antiretroviral therapy and home-based care below.

Chapter 4

Policy Options

Given the evidence of the interactions, what options exist for responding to the HIV/AIDS–food-insecurity nexus? The rationale here is twofold—first, to raise the chances that food and nutrition security policies and programs can achieve their original objectives despite AIDS, and, second, to contribute to the multisectoral response to HIV/AIDS.

First we briefly review current policy aimed at combating food and nutrition insecurity. The past few years have seen a renewed international emphasis on these outcomes (or, relatedly, on "hunger"), spurred in large part by the Millennium Development Goals (MDGs). Primary among these is the goal to halve hunger by 2015. Several important stocktaking and visioning exercises have been conducted, including the Millennium Project Hunger Task Force's recommendations (Millennium Project 2004), a new (UK) Department for International Development policy paper (DFID 2003a) and subsequent electronic consultation on "New Directions for Agriculture in Reducing Poverty," the IFPRI 2020 Vision Conference "A Way Forward from the 2020 Africa Conference: Assuring Food and Nutrition Security in Africa by 2020" (IFPRI 2004), and the U.S. Presidential Initiative to End Hunger in Africa (IEHA). Taken together, these recommendations point to a clear consensus on key action priorities:

Rural livelihoods. Increase agricultural productivity of food-insecure farmers, particularly smallholders. Increase income for the food-insecure through both farm and nonfarm livelihoods. Make markets work for the poor; improve access and infrastructure, such as roads.

Social protection. Reduce risk and vulnerability through appropriate safety nets and, where required, food aid.

Nutrition and human capital. Improve the nutritional status of vulnerable groups. Ensure public-health and education policies that support the poor, especially girls and women.

Governance and capacity. Foster good governance and public accountability, and develop capacity.

In this section, reviewing these policy instruments through an HIV/AIDS lens, we continue to follow the logic and left-to-right flow of Figure 1. We thus start with nutrition and human capital, including the specific issue of support for orphans and vulnerable children (OVCs), before focusing on safety nets in general and the role of food aid. We then look at rural livelihoods, particularly those deriving from agriculture, before turning to the overriding issue of women's empowerment and gender equity. In each of these discussions, we suggest ways in which policies may need to change to improve their HIV responsiveness, based as far as possible on the limited but growing evidence.

There is no magic bullet. Antiretroviral drugs, for example, are certainly not a universal panacea (as we discuss below). There are real dangers in generalization (Jayne et al. 2003): in agriculture, for example, such factors as ratios of land, capital, and labor and the relative degree of substitutability among household resources will determine the nature and scope of possible responses to HIV/AIDS. This all cautions against any form of blueprint response to interactions between HIV/AIDS and food security. One size absolutely does *not* fit all; but nor should everything necessarily have to change. The lens can help policymakers and program managers decide what needs to be done in the specific situations they confront.

We conclude here by outlining some examples of the policy options that may emerge from such a review. The responses may be undertaken by, or targeted at, individuals, households, communities, and local or national governments.

Women's Nutrition and Prevention of Mother-to-Child Transmission (MTCT) of HIV

Global estimates among breastfeeding populations show that, on average, 63 percent of children of HIV-positive mothers will not be infected by HIV; 7 percent will be infected during pregnancy, 15 percent during delivery, and 15 percent during the first two years of breastfeeding. Interventions that enhance immune function may significantly reduce transmission risks. Micronutrients may improve epithelial integrity and thus reduce risk. Evidence from human studies of subjects of unknown HIV status in Tanzania and Bangladesh suggest that antioxidants (especially vitamin E), taken during late pregnancy and early lactation, may be important in reducing the risk of subclinical mastitis (Filteau et al. 1999). Vitamin A and zinc supplementation trials in India and Bangladesh have resulted in improved gastrointestinal barrier function (Fawzi et al. 1993; Black 1998; McCullough et al. 1999; Roy et al. 1992).

Impact of Micronutrient Supplementation of Pregnant and Lactating Women on Pregnancy and Child Outcomes

Prenatal micronutrient supplementation improves pregnancy and birth outcomes. In Malawi, vitamin A supplementation in HIV-positive pregnant women lowered the risk of low birth weight (LBW) by 30 percent, improved neonatal growth rates, and reduced anemia among infants (Kumwenda et al. 2002). In South Africa, vitamin A supplementation in HIV-positive pregnant women reduced the risk of prematurity by 34 percent but had no effect on LBW (Coutsoudis et al. 1999). In a trial in Tanzania, multivitamin supplementation (including folate, thiamine, riboflavin, niacin, and vitamins B6, B12, C, and E, but not A) resulted in approximately 40 percent reductions in fetal loss, LBW, and severe preterm birth. Multivitamins (but not vitamin A) also increased CD4 and CD8 cell counts (Fawzi et al. 1998). In Zimbabwe, Friis et al. (2004) found that multimicronutrient supplementation significantly increased size at birth.

Among lactating mothers, multivitamin supplementation was also seen to lower mortality, reduce the risk of diarrhea, and improve the CD4 counts in breastfeeding infants. Maternal vitamin A supplementation reduced the risk that a breastfeeding child would develop a cough with a rapid respiratory rate, a proxy for pneumonia (Fawzi et al. 2003).

Impact of Micronutrient Supplementation of Pregnant and Lactating Women on MTCT

Results of trials to investigate whether vitamin A supplementation can reduce MTCT have been disappointing. Trials among pregnant women in Malawi and South Africa did not reduce the risk of in utero, intrapartum, or early breastfeeding transmission (Kumwenda et al. 2002; Coutsoudis et al. 1999). In Tanzania, neither multivitamin nor vitamin A supplementation of pregnant women lowered the risk of MTCT (Fawzi et al. 2000). Results of a multivitamin (B, C, and E) supplementation trial in Tanzania on MTCT during breastfeeding are, however, encouraging: modest reductions in HIV transmission through breastfeeding were achieved, and these reductions were significant among lactating mothers with compromised immunological and nutritional status. Mortality among HIV-negative children was reduced, and HIV-free survival was significantly prolonged among children born to women with impaired immunological or nutritional status. Supplementation of lactating women with vitamin A, however, increased the risk of vertical transmission in Tanzania (Fawzi et al. 2002a).

In sum, micronutrient supplementation (with both vitamin A and multivitamins) of pregnant women may improve pregnancy and birth outcomes, but there is no convincing evidence that micronutrient supplementation (with either vitamin A or multivitamins) during pregnancy reduces the risk of MTCT in utero, intrapartum, or during early breastfeeding. Multivitamin supplementation during lactation (with vitamins B, C, and E, not A), on the other hand, may reduce MTCT through breastfeeding, especially among women with compromised immunological and nutritional status.

Most trials began supplementation at the first prenatal visit, at approximately 20 weeks of gestation. Whether micronutrient supplementation needs to be started prepregnancy or early in pregnancy to have an impact on MTCT in utero and intrapartum is not yet known. It is therefore critical that *all women of childbearing age in areas where rapid HIV spread and malnutrition coexist—particularly poor, pregnant, and lactating women—maintain adequate nutritional status.*

Infant Feeding and Prevention of MTCT

Nowhere is the influence of HIV/AIDS on policy more dramatic than in the issue of MTCT, where the finding that HIV is transmitted through breast milk has seriously complicated infant feeding recommendations. The latest guidelines (WHO 2001) state:

> When replacement feeding is acceptable, feasible, affordable, sustainable, and safe, avoidance of all breastfeeding by HIV-infected mothers is recommended. Otherwise exclusive breastfeeding is recommended during the first months of life. To minimize HIV transmission risk, breastfeeding should be discontinued as soon as feasible, taking into account local circumstances, the individual women's situation and the risks of replacement feeding (including infections other than HIV and malnutrition).

Much of the early, often rancorous debate in this area has revealed a limited understanding of the multiple extra benefits of exclusive breastfeeding and the potential dangers of moving away from such a policy recommendation without serious assessment of the other risks. The Global Burden of Disease study (Caulfield et al. 2004), for example, states that 60 percent of child mortality (that is, 3.7 million deaths among children under five every year), is associated with malnutrition, a large proportion of which is related to poor infant feeding (including nonexclusive breastfeeding during the first six months).

The overriding question is, what is safest for child and mother? Unfortunately, there is no simple answer. Many additional issues need to be addressed concerning the numerous risk factors in breastfeeding and replacement feeding.

The risk of viral transmission through breastfeeding from an HIV-positive mother is determined by a mix of maternal and infant risk factors. Maternal risk factors include a mother's immune status, her HIV viral load, the viral concentration in her breast milk, whether she has, or is prone to, breast infections (such as mastitis), and the characteristics of the specific virus with which she has been infected. Child risk factors include duration of breastfeeding, nonexclusive breastfeeding, age, presence of mouth or intestinal lesions, prematurity, and infant immune response.

Regarding replacement feeding as the alternative, what defines "acceptable, feasible, affordable, sustainable and safe"?

A recent review by Coutsoudis and Rollins (2003) squarely confronts this dilemma and concludes that, although breastfeeding carries greater risk of mother-to-child-transmission of HIV, replacement feeding in developing countries carries an increased risk for infant mortality. This is borne out by a recent modeling exercise by Ross and Labbock (2004), which showed that six months of exclusive breastfeeding is less risky than replacement feeding for many HIV-infected women. Compared with artificial feeding, breastfeeding during the first six months by HIV-positive mothers increases HIV-free survival by 32 per 1,000 live births; after six months, as the age-specific mortality rate and risk of death caused by replacement feeding both decline, replacement feeding appears to be safer. While calling for a balanced view of the risks and full support to enable mothers to make an informed choice, Coutsoudis and Rollins (2003) point out the stark reality: without free infant formula, most HIV-infected women will choose breastfeeding for socioeconomic and cultural reasons. The onus therefore is on health workers and policymakers to make infant feeding safer.

One step forward would be to reframe the debate so as to focus on the broader, more appropriate, and less emotionally charged issue of how to maximize child survival, not just how to reduce HIV transmission through breastfeeding. Keeping HIV-positive mothers healthy and well-nourished may be the single most important, and until recently the most neglected, goal.

Nutritional Counseling, Care, and Support of the Individual Living with HIV/AIDS

For individuals living with HIV/AIDS, nutritional counseling, care, and support are necessary to put the brakes on the vicious cycle in Figure 3. Nutritional support can prolong the asymptomatic period of relative health, forestall the onset of debilitating and life-threatening opportunistic diseases (such as diarrhea, pneumonia, and tuberculosis), and ultimately prolong the lives of individuals, for their own benefit and that of young children who depend on them (Piwoz and Preble 2000). Energy requirements are raised by 10 to 30 percent following HIV infection in adults and by 50 to 100 percent among children experiencing weight loss.[4] It is thus essential that those who are infected have access to diets of adequate quality, and quantity.

The main nutrition interventions are counseling on specific behaviors, prescribed and targeted nutrition supplements, and linkages with food-based interventions and programs (Piwoz 2004). Three different types of nutrition supplements may be considered: food rations to counter mild weight loss and the nutrition-related side effects of antiretroviral drug (ARV) therapy and to address nutritional needs in food-insecure areas; micronutrient supplements for specific HIV-positive risk groups; and therapeutic foods for rehabilitation of moderate and severe malnutrition in HIV-positive adults and children.

Nutrition interventions can improve nutritional status of people living with HIV/AIDS. In the Tufts Nutrition for Healthy Living Study in Boston, researchers also found that body weight, fat-free mass, and BMI improved in people receiving nutritional intervention compared with those receiving a placebo (Tang 2003).

Among HIV-positive pregnant women, multivitamin supplementation (with vitamins B, C, and E) in Tanzania was shown to significantly increase CD4 and CD8 cell counts and hemoglobin levels (Fawzi et al. 1998). In Canada, vitamin C and E supplementation for three months resulted in decreased viral load in HIV-positive individuals (Allard et al. 1998). But in Zambia, short-duration multiple micronutrient supplementation (vitamins A, C, and E, and selenium and zinc) of HIV-positive individuals for two weeks did not affect CD4 cell count or hematological parameters (Kelly et al. 1999).

Vitamin A supplementation trials in the United States, South Africa, and Tanzania have not yielded promising results in terms of decreasing viral load or improving immunological status among HIV-positive individuals (Semba et al. 1998; Coutsoudis et al. 1997; Fawzi et al. 1998).

In a pathbreaking study of the effects of multivitamin supplements on HIV disease progression and mortality, Fawzi et al. (2004) compared the effects of daily supplements of preformed vitamin A and beta-carotene, multivitamins (B, C, and E), or both on the progression of HIV disease in a double-blind, placebo-controlled randomized trial of 1,078 pregnant women infected with HIV in Tanzania. They found that women who were randomly assigned to receive multivitamin supplementation were less likely to progress to advanced stages of HIV disease, maintained better CD4+ T-cell counts and lower viral loads, and had lower HIV-related morbidity

[4]Energy requirements are likely to increase by 10 percent to maintain body weight and physical activity in asymptomatic HIV-infected adults and growth in asymptomatic children. During symptomatic HIV, and subsequently during AIDS, energy requirements increase by approximately 20 to 30 percent to maintain adult body weight. Energy intakes need to be increased by 50 percent to 100 percent over normal requirements in children experiencing weight loss (WHO 2003).

and mortality rates than women who received the placebo. Vitamin A appeared to reduce the effect of multivitamins and, when given alone, had some negative effects. The authors concluded: "Multivitamin supplements delay the progression of HIV disease and provide an effective, low-cost means of delaying the initiation of antiretroviral therapy in HIV-infected women" (p. 23). An accompanying editorial suggests a clear need to confirm the new findings and to evaluate the effects of multivitamins in larger populations, particularly among persons with more advanced HIV disease or more serious nutritional deficiencies (Marston and De Cock 2004).

Children, too, can benefit from micronutrient supplementation. Among preschool children suffering from HIV, morbidity and mortality could be reduced and delayed growth, malaria, and persistent diarrhea alleviated with vitamin A supplements. Results from a Tanzanian study showed that two initial doses of vitamin A (higher than standard doses, yet still within a safe range) followed by another two doses four months later led over one year to average height and weight increases of one inch and one pound respectively, compared to the average for children given a placebo. Height increases were particularly significant among HIV-positive subjects (Coutsoudis et al. 1995; Fawzi et al. 1999; Villamor et al. 2002).

Studies of high energy and protein food supplementation, however, have found that although they may result in weight gain, the weight gained is mainly fat, not lean body mass. Such supplements—if they are indeed supplements and not substituted for part of the home diet—do not prevent or reverse muscle wasting, which is the critical determinant of survival (Piwoz and Preble 2000).

Nutritional Support and Antiretroviral Therapy (ART)

Every group interviewed [in a large Nairobi slum] listed lack of food as the most likely cause of nonadherence to ARV drug therapy. One participant succinctly stated, "If you give us ARVs, please give us food, just food." There truly is irony in providing antiretroviral drugs to populations that lack access to safe water or food.

—Marston and De Cock 2004

Treatment of people living with HIV/AIDS using antiretroviral drugs may be effective in inhibiting viral replication and decreasing viral load. But nutrition is directly relevant to treatment, too—and is all the more important now that access to antiretroviral therapy is beginning, albeit painfully slowly, to expand in developing countries. Interactions between these drugs and food and nutrition can significantly influence the success of ART by affecting drug efficacy, adherence to drug regimens, and nutritional status. Management of these interactions is critical to maximizing the benefit of ART to people living with HIV/AIDS in resource-poor settings.

We are only beginning to learn how and to what degree drug efficacy may be compromised by poor nutritional status. We know that certain antiretroviral drugs impede food absorption, metabolism, nutrient distribution, and excretion, and we know in turn that certain foods affect these aspects of drug assimilation.

Antiretroviral Therapy and Nutritional Status

Use of ARVs can improve nutritional status. Children who are treated with nucleoside analogue reverse transcriptase inhibitors (NRTIs) show a temporary increase in weight gain and linear growth rate. Highly active antiretroviral therapy (HAART) treatment leading to a reduction of the viral load to less than 500 copies/mL and to an increase in the $CD4^{+}$ counts has been shown to have a positive influence on child growth. Increases in BMI were seen only in children at an advanced stage of disease progression and poor nutritional status at the baseline (Verweel et al. 2002). In adults, ART is associated with a sustained weight gain and increased BMI (Silva et al. 1998; Schwenk et al. 1999) and with reduced anemia prevalence among injecting drug users (Semba et al. 2001). HAART has been shown to decrease the prevalence of vitamin B12, folate, selenium, and zinc deficiencies (Remacha 2003; Rousseau et al. 2000). Yet wasting—which remains predictive of clinical outcomes—is still significant among people on ART (Wanke et al. 2000).

Food, Nutrition, and Drug Efficacy

Food affects the efficacy of drug metabolism and therefore of ART. A high-fat meal increases the bioavailability of certain drugs (such as NRTIs and reverse transcriptase inhibitors), whereas a diet high in macronutrients inhibits the bioavailability of other drugs (such as protease inhibitor [PI] indinavar) (Castleman et al. 2003; WHO 2002). Many protease inhibitors, for example, must be taken on an empty stomach to allow efficient absorption. Proper absorption of protease inhibitors results in the interruption of a key step in viral replication, thus yielding noninfectious HIV particles (Yeh et al. 1998). Other drugs (such as NRTI didanosine) should be taken 30 minutes before a meal, as food reduces absorption (Castleman et al. 2003; WHO 2002). ART management should therefore be drug-specific. Zinc supplements given with zidovudine (AZT) in stage-4 HIV were associated with a 50 percent decline in opportunistic infections and an increase in zinc-bound thymulin levels, which are critical for differentiation of T-cells (Mocchegiani and Muzzioli 2000).

ARV Side Effects

Administration of ARVs is associated with metabolic alterations. Their use has been associated with a form of fat redistribution called lipodystrophy, in which central adiposity is accompanied by subcutaneous loss of fat (McDermott et al. 2001; Carr et al. 1998; Lipsky 1998). Lipodystrophy prevalence increases with duration of ARV treatment (Chen et al. 2002). Use of protease inhibitors has been associated with reduced bone mineral content among men, raising the risk of osteoporosis (McDermott et al. 2001) and increases in anthrogenic lipoproteins, plasma cholesterol, and insulin resistance, with implications for chronic disease burden such as heart disease and diabetes mellitus (Cheseaux et al. 2002). Treatment with NRTIs can lead to lactic acidosis. Nonnucleoside reverse transcriptase inhibitors (NNRTIs) and protease inhibitors are associated with cases of transaminitis and hepatotoxicity. Diabetes mellitus and insulin resistance due to ART use have also been reported (Montessori et al. 2004).

Drug side effects such as nausea, taste changes, and loss of appetite may reduce food consumption, and diarrhea and vomiting may increase nutrient losses. In a U.S. study, Chen et al. (2002) found that one in four patients who stopped ART did so because of nausea or vomiting, and these signs tended to develop early in the treatment. A Botswana study (Weiser et al. 2003) found 10 percent nonadherence due to side effects (though by far the greatest constraint, causing 44 percent of all curtailed therapy, was financial).

Most of these studies were conducted in developed countries. The implications for drug efficacy and side effects in countries with widespread malnutrition are not well understood. We found no studies investigating whether preexisting malnutrition inhibits drug bioavailability or increases side effects. And we still do not know enough about the effect of ARVs on milk composition in malnourished lactating women or how ARVs interact with specific micronutrient deficiencies.

There is, however, ample evidence that people living with HIV/AIDS in resource-limited settings are unlikely to be able to follow food and nutrition recommendations for ARV therapy because of lack of access to required foods or because they are already malnourished. Such difficulties may reduce drug adherence, a major problem in all ARV programs. Research shows that nearly 25 percent of individuals using ARVs in developed countries discontinue their treatment regimen because of treatment failure of some sort (Montessori et al. 2004). Nonadherence increases the potential for drug resistance (Jones and Holloman 2000), which in turn decreases quality of life as a result of substantial decline in health, increased frequency of opportunistic diseases, and faster progression of the disease. The risks are serious.

Another, poorly understood problem with ART is that the majority of HIV-infected individuals are not eligible for treatment with ARVs, even if the drugs are available and affordable. Available data continue to support the practice of starting therapy in asymptomatic patients when CD4+ cell counts are between 200 cells/μL and 350 cells/μL (Tomkins 2004; Saag 2004; Pallela et al. 2003). As well as being extremely important during treatment, therefore, nutritional support has potential for prolonging the period of time *before* treatment becomes necessary. Guidelines for this group are needed. One country taking a leading role is Uganda. Here, the National AIDS Control Program (NACP) is leading an inclusive, multisectoral process to develop and apply national guidelines for providing nutritional care and support to PLWHAs. The purpose is to provide policymakers, programs, caregivers, and PLWHAs with sound guidance to improve the nutritional status of those infected by HIV/AIDS.

The growing impact of the epidemic has shown that promotion of simple but important food-security, nutrition, and public-health interventions alongside and as a part of HIV/AIDS treatment initiatives is critical to an effective HIV/AIDS response. Home-based care (HBC) initiatives need to be holistic and extend beyond the person infected by HIV to include family and household members. HBC programs are shifting from an exclusive focus on medical and nursing care to include counseling, food assistance, welfare support, school fees for orphans, and income generation for widows. But capacity is severely limited: most of these programs depend on overburdened female community volunteers, and government involvement is limited (UNAIDS 2004).

Table 3 from Piwoz (2004) provides a useful summary of possible nutrition interventions according to stage of HIV disease progression.

Protecting Orphans and Vulnerable Children (OVCs)

Among the most devastating effects of the HIV/AIDS pandemic in sub-Saharan Africa is the rapidly growing orphan population. An estimated 12.3 million children in the region have been orphaned by AIDS, and this population will increase in the next decade as HIV-positive parents become ill and die. And although sub-Saharan Africa has the highest proportion of children who are orphans, the absolute numbers of orphans are much higher in Asia, which had 87.6 million orphans (from all causes) in 2003, twice the number in sub-Saharan Africa (UNAIDS/UNICEF/USAID 2004).

As well as orphans, there are millions more vulnerable children who are caring for infected family members, dropping out of school because of a lack of financial support, and going hungry or undernourished. Although traditional networks of support have been successfully caring for OVCs, their capacity has been overwhelmed by the escalating numbers of children in need. The following section outlines current strategies to improve the well-being, nutritional status, and future development of affected children in the region.

Deininger et al. (2003) suggest that the impact of the OVC crisis can be mitigated through appropriate sectoral policies. Most orphaned children in Africa are being fostered by relatives, and this seems to be the most desirable first line of response.

Table 3 Summary of nutrition interventions according to HIV disease progression

Intervention	HIV-positive, asymptomatic	HIV-positive, symptomatic	AIDS	Families affected by an HIV-related death
Counseling and care	Nutrition education and counseling for positive living	Nutrition management of HIV-related opportunistic infections (OI), symptoms, and medications	Nutrition management of antiretroviral therapy (where available) Nutrition management in home-, clinic-, and community-based palliative care	Counseling on special food and nutritional needs of orphans, vulnerable infants, and young children
Prescribed or targeted nutrition supplementation	For high-risk groups only (e.g., pregnant and lactating HIV-positive women, HIV-exposed, nonbreastfed children)	For high-risk groups For persons who are losing weight or do not respond to medications Therapeutic feeding for moderately and severely malnourished HIV-positive adults and children	Therapeutic feeding for moderately and severely malnourished HIV-positive adults and children	For high-risk groups (e.g., HIV-exposed, non-breastfed children under 2 years of age and HIV-exposed children with growth faltering)
Other food interventions	To prevent nutritional deterioration for HIV-affected families living in highly food-insecure communities	To improve adherence and participation in OI treatment programs	To improve adherence and participation in ARV and OI treatment programs To use in home-, clinic-, and community-based care programs	To protect the health of orphans and vulnerable children and for surviving family members when livelihoods are compromised because of HIV-related sickness or death

Source Piwoz 2004.

Most recommendations focus on building on existing structures within communities, such as self-help groups, women's groups, and church groups (Nyambedha et al. 2001). Little work has been done, however, in detailing specific strategies and interventions that would make such an approach feasible and sustainable for institutions already facing increased stress and diminishing resources. Sectoral policy needs to be much more proactively geared to assisting households in managing this increased burden and providing other options when capacity is exceeded.

Schooling support is critically important. Nyambedha et al. (2001) recommend that immediate action be taken to formulate and implement policies for the sustainable schooling of orphans, which has been seriously threatened in recent years by AIDS. Food-for-education programs hold great promise. The link between education, food security, and nutrition is not direct, but it is very significant (Smith and Haddad 2000). Children who are fed in schools are more likely to attend school, less likely to drop out, and better able to learn. As educated individuals, they face better future prospects, and the prospects of their own children are also enhanced. HIV/AIDS prevention education may also be delivered at school (Ainsworth and Filmer 2002).

Providing incentives for children to attend school through school feeding and support for, or waiving of, school fees is thus an important policy goal. Deininger et al. (2003) showed that after the adoption of universal primary education in Uganda in 1997, being a foster child no longer impeded access to education. In the absence of proactive policies, however, young foster children's access to health services worsened over time. School feeding has been seen to keep children in school in Zimbabwe. In a study of food-insecure households, 25 percent of children had dropped out of nonfeeding schools in the previous year, compared to 15 percent where school feeding was in place (SADC FANR 2003).

Box 4. Case studies of OVC initiatives

Scaling Up HIV/AIDS Interventions through Expanded Partnerships (STEPs) in Malawi. STEPs is a community-driven approach to scaling up HIV/AIDS interventions. Supported by USAID and Save the Children U.S. (SC), STEPs started in 1995 (then called COPE, Community-based Options for Protection and Empowerment) as a service-delivery program in one district in Malawi to assist children affected by HIV/AIDS. Through evaluations, SC realized such an approach was not sustainable, cost-effective, or scalable. On the basis of recommendations from the evaluations and the field experience, the program revitalized the dormant decentralized AIDS committees (at the district, community, and village levels) and their technical subcommittees under the National AIDS Commission (NAC), in the Namwera community in Mangochi to mobilize collective action to combat the epidemic.

Based in turn on the positive experience in Namwera, the program changed its initial strategy to that of an external agent for change, assisting communities with community mobilization and capacity building so that communities become empowered to act collectively to address their own problems. Village AIDS Committees (VACs) identify the vulnerable and plan responses on the basis of the nature and magnitude of vulnerability within the villages, the needs of the vulnerable, and the capacity within the villages to respond. They also monitor the program's activities and mobilize resources. As the needs of the most affected communities are multiple, the program has evolved into a truly multisectoral program, offering prevention, care, support, and mitigation activities. STEPs has also influenced national policies related to HIV/AIDS and children. Through partnerships and training other NGOs and CBOs (community-based organizations) in the program approach of community mobilization and facilitating collective action, STEPs and similar models aim to cover 75 percent of Malawi's population (Kadiyala 2004).

CHIN in Zambia. In Zambia, the government, NGOs, and UNICEF have collaborated to establish the Children in Need Network (CHIN). CHIN provides support to registered NGOs and CBOs working with vulnerable children (www.chin.org.zm). Although the organization does not directly provide food aid or nutritional support, it works to promote and foster economic empowerment for households through programs, training, and income-generating activities so that families who have taken in orphans are better equipped to handle the increased economic burden.

Community-based child-care centers in Nthondo, Malawi. World Vision assisted the Nthondo community members to pool their resources and donate their time and effort to establish and run 10 child-care centers catering to about 335 boys and 326 girls. Local leaders have also donated farmland on which to establish community gardens. School volunteers, in collaboration with the local leaders, mobilize people in the surrounding villages to work on the gardens. Produce from the gardens is used to feed the children in the centers, with leftover produce being sold at the local market to help meet the running costs of the centers.

Indlunkhulu in Swaziland. The word *indlunkhulu* refers to the tradition of distributing food from the chief's fields to members of the community who are unable to support themselves. In Swazi law and custom, chiefs are responsible for the welfare of orphans within their area. This practice provides an existing basis on which to build a sustainable mechanism for the delivery of food to orphans and vulnerable children. The implementing agency for the Indlunkhulu project is the Ministry of Agriculture and Cooperatives. Through the Ministry, the National Emergency Response Committee on HIV/AIDS (NERCHA) provided the initial agricultural inputs for the Indlunkhulu fields. Community members plow and tend the crops. OVCs also assist in tilling the fields; this gives them practical experience in subsistence farming, helping them to develop skills for later in life. The Indlunkhulu fields are intended to provide a sustainable source of food for OVCs.

Ainsworth and Semali (2000) in Tanzania found that immunization against measles, oral rehydration therapy, and improved access to health care can disproportionately improve health outcomes among poorest children, and, within that group, particularly among children affected by adult mortality. The World Bank has estimated that the cheapest alternative for recurrent support to orphans is to provide them with schooling and nutritional supplements (Deininger et al. 2003).

Another recent World Bank report (Deininger et al. 2003) has recommended different categories of OVC interventions, including a food and nutrition intervention strategy that supports food donations to informal institutions as well as the provision and delivery of food baskets to households, particularly those with young children.

The World Food Programme (WFP 2002) has outlined a number of policy interventions aimed at providing food and nutritional support for OVCs, including linking up food aid and home-based care programs, food-for-training opportunities for older children, and school feeding programs at both elementary and preschool levels to alleviate short-term hunger and provide a better learning environment.

Drawing on lessons learned, an important multiorganizational framework for the protection, care, and support of OVCs has recently been published (UNAIDS/UNICEF 2004). Its key strategies are:

- strengthen the capacity of families to protect and care for orphans and vulnerable children by prolonging the lives of parents and providing economic, psychosocial, and other support;
- mobilize and support community-based responses;
- ensure access for orphans and vulnerable children to essential services, including birth registration, education, and health care;
- ensure that governments protect the most vulnerable children through improved policy and legislation and by channeling resources to families and communities; and
- raise awareness at all levels through advocacy and social mobilization to create a supportive environment for children and families affected by HIV/AIDS.

NGOs in particular are playing an important role in establishing intervention policy and practices. For example, the STEPs program (see Box 4) is working with 20,000 orphans in Malawi to mobilize and conduct care and support activities, providing food security, education, and psychosocial assistance as well as working to assist families caring for OVCs.

Overall, however, the response remains inadequate to the magnitude and continuing deterioration of the OVC situation in sub-Saharan Africa. Even in one of the more progressive countries, Uganda, for example, the combined efforts of NGOs, governments, and donors currently reach only 5 percent of the 1.7 million orphans in the country.

There are very few evaluations of OVC interventions, first, because there is still an incomplete understanding of the complexities of household coping responses, local caregiving practices, and stigma, as well as a lack of data on preschool enrollment rates, the number of children caring for sick family members, and the number of child-headed households (World Bank 2003); and second, because intervention strategies are still relatively recent, and it is too early to evaluate many of them.

Ensuring Safety Nets

Many HIV/AIDS impacts are revealed through the responses adopted by individuals, households, and communities. Some of these responses are examples of resilience, but many derive from distress. The first line of defense has been communities, many of whom have responded in very innovative ways. Documented responses include labor sharing, orphan support, community-based child care, community food banks, credit schemes for funeral benefits, and new ways of reducing the time and energy required for domestic tasks, such as fuel and water collection and food preparation (Mutangadura 1999; Drimie 2003; Donovan et al. 2003; NAADS 2003).

The scope and depth of social capital and social networks often determine the viability of local responses. Interestingly, richer households are usually richer not only in physical and human capital but also in social capital: for example, in the Kagera study in Tanzania, they were more likely to receive private assistance, and they received more assistance overall than poor households (Lundberg and Over 2000). Formal sources accounted for more than a third of all financial assistance received by the poorest households a month after an adult death.

To maximize food and nutrition security in the context of HIV/AIDS, the overriding priorities should be to (1) augment community and household resistance and resilience as far as possible, and (2) ensure there are safety nets in place for those who are unable to cope otherwise. Efforts should move from an "individual-infected" model to a "community-affected" one and focus on strengthening community capacity for response. The emphasis in mitigation strategy needs to be on strengthening *resilience,* the ability of households and communities to adapt livelihood strategies that allow them to recover from the shock of HIV/AIDS. Policy needs to draw on measures already in effect in communities where proactive responses are under way. Where households and communities' capacity to cope has been exceeded, a broad-based social-security system offering minimal benefits or specifically targeted welfare programs may be important for mitigation in the short and medium term.

Nutritionally balanced food aid may also be important as a safety net for those acutely food-insecure, or at risk of becoming so. Food aid has significant potential not only for mitigating AIDS impacts on food security but also for reducing the susceptibility of people to the HIV virus by preventing the adoption of risky livelihood strategies. Table 4 provides some examples of options for effectively utilizing food

Table 4 Applying an HIV/AIDS lens to food-aid programs

Program	Design features in non-HIV context	Design features in heavy HIV/AIDS context
Income generation and microcredit	• Mostly targeted at women's groups • Difficulty in reaching ultra-poor	• Could be targeted to PLWHA associations, OVCs, and other vulnerable groups, such as elderly-headed households and households taking in foster children. • Lack of trust regarding repayment in group-based lending schemes; greater stigma and social exclusion.
Food for assets or work	• Based on the premise of labor abundance and self-targeting • Labor-intensive public works	• Labor may not be abundant, and self-targeting will not work for PLWHAs or labor-short households headed by children or elderly people, which are often least able to undertake manual work. • Dissemination of labor-saving technologies, promotion of labor and tool banks; crop diversification with an emphasis on labor-efficient and nutrient-rich crops.
Food for training	• Often limited to training volunteers, mostly health and extension workers • Used mostly in food-insecure regions	• Should be expanded to include traditional birth attendants, home-based and community-based child-care center volunteers, volunteer teachers in informal schools, and teachers to be trained in HIV/AIDS-related issues. • Could be expanded to high-prevalence areas (regardless of degree of food security at the regional level).
Food for education	• One of the most popular food-aid interventions, mostly targeting schools in chronically food-insecure regions • Extra take-home ration given to girls	• Could be expanded to areas of high HIV prevalence, regardless of food security at the regional level. • Extra take-home ration could be given not only to girls but also to OVCs. Involvement of the community is crucial to prevent stigma of OVCs.
Food for health	• Supplementary feeding of pregnant women • No attention paid to adult illness	• Supplementary feeding of pregnant women and support of HIV-positive mothers and their infants. • Critical to provide nutrition interventions to chronically ill through home-based care.

Table 4—Continued

Program	Design features in non-HIV context	Design features in heavy HIV/AIDS context
Food for life (emergency response)	• Often limited to distribution of relief food • Characterized by food-centered response • No special attention to youth • Little attention paid to often dismal living conditions of host populations around refugee camps	• Need for structural response to build capacity and livelihoods, to prevent survival sex and exploitative power relations. • Need for nutrition response with special attention to chronically ill and pregnant and lactating women. • Crucial to containing the epidemic. Need for strategies to assist youth, especially girls, in negotiating safe sexual practices and livelihood approaches. • Exploitation of refugees by host population and vice versa is prevalent and fuels the epidemic. Investments in improving livelihoods and HIV-relevant education of *all* population groups should be given priority.

Source: Kadiyala and Gillespie 2004.

assistance, not only as a safety net but also to leverage livelihood opportunities (Kadiyala and Gillespie 2004).

With regard to managing the coexistence of acute food insecurity and high HIV prevalence, a three-pronged attack has been recommended (SADC FANR 2003):

1. *Consumption-side support.* Chronic illness of the head of household and the presence of an elderly head of household, in particular a woman, cross-checked with a wealth-group analysis, are useful indicators for targeting food aid. But agencies will need to work with communities to ensure that AIDS-affected households are not excluded. School feeding programs have the combined benefits of ensuring that more children consume a healthy meal at least once per day, reducing the dropout rate, promoting education and empowerment, and reducing the time children spend unsupervised—especially young girls, who may be at risk of increased exposure to HIV.
2. *Productivity-enhancing support.* This includes rapid introduction of interventions with a high food-access-to-labor ratio that are accessible to AIDS-affected households.
3. *Household and community safety nets.* These may include services to support micro enterprises, savings schemes, and community resource mobilization involving strengthening of social capital, and fund-raising.

There is a need for a paradigm shift from the approach of a sequential continuum of care—from relief to rehabilitation to development—toward the *contiguum* approach, which recognizes that all these approaches are interrelated, and any one of them may be needed at any time. In this context, a recent high-level United Nations report has recommended a dual approach of "emergency development" and "developmental relief," essentially combining urgent humanitarian assistance with a longer-term, capacity-strengthening response aimed at sustainable development (United Nations 2004).

Supporting Livelihoods

Agriculture-Based Livelihoods

The main source of livelihood for most people affected by HIV/AIDS is agriculture. There is tremendous scope for agricultural policy to become more HIV-responsive not only in order to further AIDS-related objectives but also, crucially, to ensure that its own objectives remain achievable.

In order to offset increasing labor constraints, labor and time management may be facilitated through:

- increasing access, particularly for poor women, to labor-saving technologies (for example, lightweight plows, fuel-efficient stoves, water-pumping systems, grinding mills, and dehuskers);
- smoothing peaks and bottlenecks in labor demand; and
- reducing the labor requirements of systems of cropping (e.g., through improved seed varieties, zero- or minimum-tillage techniques, and intercropping), soil conservation (e.g., using soil-holding grasses, not labor-intensive ridging), animal husbandry (e.g., rearing smaller stock, such as poultry), pest control (e.g., using trap crops to attract pests away from crops), and postharvest storage (Jayne et al. 2003).

Options and incentives for improving diets (such as keeping home gardens and raising poultry and small livestock) and ensuring diversity and nutritional quality of food crops (for example, orange-fleshed sweet potatoes, beans, and peas) can be explored, particularly working through NGOs and CBOs to develop community-level demonstration sites.

Though few have been evaluated and most are small-scale, an increasing number of HIV-responsive agricultural interventions are being implemented. Examples include conservation farming, tractor-hire services, and postharvest and processing technologies in the Bondo and Busia districts of Kenya (Bishop-Sambrook 2003), agricultural support and training, vocational training, and provision of credit and

Box 5. Drip irrigation in Zimbabwe

A small USAID-funded pilot project—poised to expand rapidly across Zimbabwe—provides AIDS-affected families with simple drip-irrigation kits for household gardens, giving them a chance to improve their nutritional intake and increase their income by growing vegetables for consumption and sale. Working through 10 NGOs, International Development Enterprises (IDE) produces and distributes kits that can irrigate a household garden of up to 100 square meters, cutting irrigation labor requirements by half. At a cost of US $85 IDE can provide one irrigation kit with a stand, fencing for the garden, training, information, and follow-up support. Five hundred kits have been installed thus far; 20,000 could rapidly be placed with AIDS-affected households through the existing NGO network.

loan schemes in Uganda, Tanzania, Lesotho, and Zimbabwe (White 2002), pit farming in Zambia[5] (Connolly 2003), and community grain banks in Malawi (Connolly 2003). Box 5 highlights an innovation from Zimbabwe. Other projects have focused on the promotion of agrobiodiversity and indigenous knowledge (Du Guerny 2002; Gari and Villareal 2002).

Constraints on the adoption of new technologies include lack of knowledge, information, cash, and time; a weak bargaining position; isolation of those affected; attitudes; and tradition. New technologies require inputs, time, and knowledge in the short term to become effective (Bishop-Sambrook 2003). The author identifies three domains for action: to increase farmers' exposure to new ideas and access to information; to develop skills and attitudes that permit the sustained use of labor-saving technologies and practices; and to increase farmers' access to relevant technologies.

Agricultural knowledge can be preserved through the development of HIV-aware and gender-proactive agricultural extension capacity. "Farmer field and life schools," successfully implemented in Cambodia, could be developed. In the field school, men and women farmers learn through field observations, discussions, and analysis of issues like crop management and income-generating activities. The life school uses a similar process to strengthen men's and women's understanding of how their socioeconomic vulnerability leads to risky behavior and tries to establish

[5]Pit farming involves digging round holes and then filling them with a mixture of organic material (household trash, crop residues, animal manure, and topsoil) for composting over a period of two to three months. Crops are then planted under monoculture or mixed-cropping conditions. Holes can be used for four to five years before they need to be refilled with organic material. Some farmers intercrop legumes, such as cowpeas or groundnuts, with maize or sorghum in their pits. This method of crop production is categorized as "conservation tillage" and conserves water and labor (as it requires minimal cultivation and weeding).

Table 5 Applying an HIV/AIDS lens to subsistence agricultural policy

Susceptibility	Vulnerability
Assessment	
• What is the known HIV prevalence? • Are multiple sexual partners common? • Is there occasional or regular migration for wage work? • Are there high levels of alcohol consumption? • What is the proximity to transport or trading centers? • Are there frequent interactions with market centers? • Is the status of women low? • Do women have limited economic independence? • Are there major economic differentials between men and women? • Are physically damaging sexual practices employed? • Is there widespread exchange of cash or favors for sexual services?	• How prevalent are poverty, malnutrition, and food insecurity? • Is the climate dry? • What are the rainfall patterns? • Is the range of crops limited? • Are there marked labor peaks in the agricultural cycle? • Are there very labor-intensive agricultural processes? • Do households exchange labor? • Are there conflicts between domestic and farming tasks? • Is it possible to replace existing labor-intensive food crops with less labor-demanding ones? • Are food surpluses adequate? • Are there opportunities for off-farm income? • Is land tenure secure or insecure?
Action	
• Increase locally generated incomes and thus reduce the need to migrate for work • Develop support groups for women and men to discuss sexual health • Integrate information about the longer-term impacts of HIV/AIDS on household income and welfare into extension programs • Encourage and support programs promoting education on safer sex, affordable, available, and effective diagnosis and treatment of STDs, availability of affordable condoms, access to safe nonsexual recreations (particularly for adolescents); increasing the economic independence of women; and reducing alcohol consumption	• Classify farming systems according to vulnerability to the impact of increased illness and death • Explore labor-efficient crop varieties • Explore introduction of small livestock to supplement protein intake • Explore labor-efficient cultivation practices—for example, development and improvement of intercropping • Explore ways of reducing women's work burden—for example, labor-efficient methods of preparing food and obtaining water and fuel • Explore introduction of simple labor-saving cultivation technologies—for example, hand tillers and draft animals • Explore ways of reducing postharvest losses • Use paddocking for larger stock to reduce herding labor
Actions that may reduce both susceptibility and vulnerability	
• Encourage labor exchanges between households • Educate orphaned children in local farming techniques • Integrate sexual-health education with agricultural-extension messages • Review land tenure arrangements to protect the occupancy and inheritance rights of widows and orphaned children	

Source: Adapted from USAID 2000.

a farmers' network to address local issues. Opportunities could also be sought for incorporating agriculture in the school curricula. Capacity constraints may be mitigated through better communications, such as rural radio.

The competitiveness and productivity of smallholder agriculture can be supported through increased public investment in transport and communications infrastructure and the development of markets for secure land rental and for local sale of products (Jayne et al. 2003).

Agriculture policy should consider generating new incentives for collective action and the formation and preservation of social capital so as to enable the protection of common property resources, such as rangelands, river basins, and forests. Tree planting and preservation, for example, may be considered to preserve the soil quality of fallow land.

HIV/AIDS prevention is conventionally equated with sex education, condom distribution, and behavioral change. But opening up opportunities for less risky, less susceptible livelihoods also constitutes prevention: for example, diversifying livelihoods to ensure food and nutrition security may preclude the need for an adult to migrate for work and help keep families together. Within commercial agriculture, encouraging "safe migration" by providing incentives for families to move together to places where work is available will be important. Table 5 provides an illustration of the questions and options that might flow from applying an HIV/AIDS lens to subsistence agriculture, differentiating susceptibility to HIV spread from vulnerability to AIDS impacts. Table 6 takes the example of the recently released Ugandan Food and Nutrition Policy (Government of Uganda 2003) and applies the lens to some of its different policy instruments.

Microfinance

In the context of HIV/AIDS, microfinance—the tailoring of financial services to the needs of low-income households—may have the following limitations: (1) it is usually small-scale, currently serving only about two million clients across Africa; (2) there is an inherent tension between scale (the number of clients served) and the extent of services provided to the clients; and (3) it often cannot serve the neediest, who are most likely to default on loans (Parker et al. 2000). Affected households may find it difficult to position themselves in a competitive market. In Zimbabwe, for example, HIV-affected households undertaking microenterprises experienced a decline in profits compared to other households between 1997 and 1999 (Barnes et al. 2001).

Microfinance does have potential for helping mitigate the socioeconomic impacts of AIDS (see Box 6). Innovations include mandatory loan-default insurance, mandatory death-benefit insurance, legal services, and the provision of education trusts for children.

Table 6 Reviewing the Uganda Food and Nutrition Policy through an HIV/AIDS lens

Policy instrument	How policy instrument might interact with HIV/AIDS	How policy instrument might be modified or supplemented to address this interaction
Section 3.1.2, objective (i): To promote and diversify the production of food commodities to meet the nutritional needs of households.	Those affected may be less likely to diversify because of labor and time constraints in HIV/AIDS-affected households. Households often resort to low-input, low-output crop production that tends to be lower in nutritious value.	Promote agro-forestry; provide nutrition education to make best use of locally available foods. Train youth in growing diversified crops and raising small livestock.
Section 3.1.2, objective (iv): To promote technologies that are appropriate to the farming systems in different agro-ecological zones.	HIV/AIDS-affected households often lack information because of isolation and lack the cash, time, and bargaining power to adopt these technologies. Often HIV/AIDS-related vulnerable groups do not benefit from these interventions.	Analyze constraints and opportunities affecting adoption of technologies by those affected by HIV/AIDS to inform technology development and dissemination.
Section 3.1.2, objective (viii): To encourage income-generating activities that improve the purchasing power of families.	These activities often require capital, and those affected by HIV/AIDS tend to have fewer assets. Women bear the double burden of producing food and caring for the sick. Marketing of goods may require travel away from home, which increases the chances of risky behaviors.	Develop innovative microcredit schemes to benefit affected households. Low-input, low- but quick-return activities may be most appropriate. Review the opening and closing times of markets. Target some activities to PLWHA associations, OVCs, and other vulnerable groups, such as elderly-headed households. Incorporate life skills training and other HIV-AIDS management-related skills, particularly where income-generating activity requires time away from community.

Section 3.1.2, objective (ix): To ensure the availability of, and access to, user-friendly credit facilities and other inputs that are essential for the modernization and commercialization of agriculture.	Microcredit does not often reach the neediest. Difficulties in loan repayment can lead to further indebtedness. Lack of trust exists regarding repayment in group-based lending in regions of high HIV prevalence; greater stigma and social exclusion can result. Vulnerable groups such as PLWHA, older people, and youth tend to be left out of such initiatives.	Allow for longer initiation time to motivate those affected by HIV/AIDS. Incorporate provision of death insurance into credit initiatives; offer health insurance for clients and families, flexible savings plans, greater flexibility on loan sizes and payment schedules, emergency loans, and HIV/AIDS awareness training. Target activities at PLWHA associations, OVCs, and other vulnerable groups, such as elderly-headed households.
Section 3.3.1, objective (iii): To develop a reliable network of appropriate food transport systems. Section 3.3.2, objective (iv): To develop and expand local and external food markets.	Proximity to road networks and markets are determinants of risky behavior that fuels the spread of HIV.	Strengthen prevention activities in such areas by providing education, condoms, and voluntary counseling and testing (VCT). Incorporate participatory approaches.
Section 3.5: To restrict food aid to the alleviation of temporary food crises and to ensure its safety for human consumption. Section 3.5.2, objective (iii): To provide food to those who cannot feed themselves for reasons beyond their control.	The number of people requiring nonemergency food aid may increase. Those most affected by HIV/AIDS, such as PLWHAs and their families, tend to require food assistance for longer following a crisis. Other vulnerable groups would include OVCs and elderly-headed households.	Use food aid (from either local reserves or external food aid) creatively to preserve or enhance the assets of those affected, build human capital (including nutrition and education), and motivate and train HBC workers.
Section 3.7.2, objective (ii): To reduce undernutrition among adolescents and women of reproductive age. Section 3.7.2, objective (iii): To reduce the incidence of low birth weight.	More women than men are HIV-positive. Those with the virus are more likely to be suffering from multiple nutrient deficiencies. HIV and malnutrition among pregnant women increase the likelihood of adverse birth outcomes. Malnutrition also increases the likelihood of mother-to-child transmission of HIV.	Promote adequate nutrition for all women. Strengthen and expand maternal supplementary feeding through MCH clinics and nutrition education.

Box 6. Case studies in microfinance

IMAGE is an innovative program in South Africa that emphasizes the importance of the environment in which sexual behaviors, gender-based violence, and HIV infections occur. It combines the introduction of a poverty-targeted microfinance program to rural communities with a participatory learning and action curriculum for clients (IMAGE 2002).

Measures undertaken by the Zambuko Trust in Zimbabwe (Barnes et al. 2001) to reduce the impact of client death on its financial portfolio include a mandatory insurance fee of 1 percent to cover the loan if the client dies, a mandatory savings requirement, a policy of loaning only to economically active persons, and strict enforcement of group coguarantees of loan installments. Comparing Zambuko Trust's HIV-affected clients to HIV-affected nonclients showed that a significantly greater proportion of boys aged six to sixteen were in school, and 16 percent more clients than nonclients had individual savings accounts with a formal institution.

Freedom from Hunger and World Relief worked together to develop a strategy that offers clients a combination of microfinance and health education. They developed a curriculum for HIV/AIDS education provided to microfinance groups during repayment meetings. The curriculum is designed for community microcredit groups using a credit-with-education methodology (whereby health and business education are offered along with credit), but it can be used by any group that meets regularly, rural or urban. Implementation started in September 2002. These organizations are currently implementing the curriculum globally in their microfinance programs.

Women's Empowerment and Human Rights

The social and economic status of women, as discussed earlier, is one of the most, possibly *the* most, important single factor conditioning the spread of HIV and the ability of households and communities to withstand its impacts. Reviewing existing approaches to address gender in HIV/AIDS-relevant programming, Gupta et al. (2003) outline a continuum of approaches that have been used:

1. interventions which, at a minimum, do no harm;
2. gender-sensitive interventions that recognize that men's and women's needs often differ and find ways to meet those needs;
3. gender-transformative interventions that not only recognize and address gender differences but also foster conditions in which women and men can examine the damaging aspects of gender norms and experiment with new behaviors to create more equitable roles and relationships; and
4. structural interventions that reduce gender inequalities by empowering women and girls. By increasing women's access to economic and social resources, such interventions can fundamentally change the economic and social dynamic of gender roles and relationships and, in the long term, protect women as well as men and families in the HIV/AIDS epidemic.

Box 7. Legal-service vouchers to protect assets in Zimbabwe

Linkages for the Economic Advancement of the Disadvantaged (LEAD), a program of Development Alternatives, Inc (DAI), cooperates with local AIDS service organizations (ASOs), HIV/AIDS-focused NGOs, and local law firms in Zimbabwe to protect the assets of targeted low-income, AIDS-affected households. It provides vouchers for legal services (such as drawing up wills and handling guardianship and maintenance claims). The LEAD program selects ASOs and AIDS-focused NGOs to educate their members on the voucher program and to issue vouchers to those who qualify. Currently the project partners with at least 11 organizations to issue vouchers. Once they have received the vouchers, clients consult a lawyer of their choice from participating law firms. The law firm provides services to the client and then submits the voucher to LEAD for payment.

Source: AED 2003.

Gender-sensitive programs may address individuals' vulnerabilities in the short term, but transformative and empowering programs ultimately are required to challenge the root causes of the epidemic (Gupta et al. 2003).

Inheritance laws and customs can have particularly negative consequences for women and for AIDS-affected households. Widows lose some or all of their assets (including their land and homes) to relatives of the deceased spouse. They are often left destitute and thus more susceptible to HIV and more vulnerable to further consequences of HIV/AIDS. In Uganda, widows were found to be reluctant to rent out land for fear of losing their rights to it (Barnett 1994).

Guaranteeing women's property and inheritance rights in the context of HIV/AIDS requires both global and national-level actions. A recent review (UNAIDS 2004) recommends action in five key areas:

1. documenting women's land and housing rights and tenure security in areas of high HIV/AIDS prevalence;
2. raising public awareness, especially among national policymakers and donors;
3. reforming legislation, including customary law and practice;
4. identifying strategic litigation opportunities, especially by improving legal skills, establishing legal precedents through test cases, improving the court system, and ensuring women's access to legal structures and processes; and
5. identifying and supporting experimentation within communities to change economic and institutional arrangements, including initiatives that support the collective ownership or lease rights to land and establishing land trusts for orphans.

Chapter 5

Scaling Up, Mainstreaming, and Capacity Development

Most HIV/AIDS prevention, care, and treatment programs are very small and have been referred to as "expensive boutiques," available only to a small percentage of the affected population (Binswanger 2000). While much can be learned from the proliferation of small-scale, innovative responses—whose successes need to be communicated more widely—it is also crucial to look for ways of effectively and fairly rapidly scaling up approaches that work in different contexts. Scaling up is not just a matter of expanding HIV program coverage; it can also involve increasing organizational involvement through mainstreaming (Gillespie 2004).

Mainstreaming is the process of harnessing and developing the capacity of an organization or sector to respond at the broadest level. It is different from integration, which may involve simply adding or linking an AIDS-specific component or intervention to another development program—or adding a chapter on AIDS to a development plan. Unlike integration, mainstreaming influences an institution's core business, possibly changing both *what* is done and *how* it is done. It is an iterative process that leads eventually to HIV/AIDS considerations being fully factored into problem assessment, causal and resource analysis, and action plans.

Stemming the spread of HIV and mitigating its impacts requires multisectoral strategies and effective mainstreaming across and within a range of development sectors. HIV epidemics are themselves multisectoral, in terms of both etiology and impact. A program's original goals may no longer be achievable unless AIDS is considered in planning and design (see Box 8). There is certainly little chance of the Millennium Development Goals (MDGs) being met in most countries in sub-Saharan Africa without a proactive focus on HIV/AIDS.

It is thus necessary to educate various sectors about the role they can play in all aspects of the response to HIV/AIDS: prevention, care, treatment, and impact mitigation. We have described use of the HIV lens for this purpose. Many frameworks, resource packs, and toolkits have been developed recently to facilitate these efforts. These include macro-level initiatives such as integrating HIV/AIDS into poverty-reduction strategy papers (PRSPs) and initiatives for highly indebted poor countries (HIPCs) (UNDP 2002); sectoral-level mainstreaming, such as the efforts to mainstream HIV/AIDS in ministries of agriculture (Topouzis 2003; Elsey et al. 2003) and the sectoral toolkits produced by the Health Economics and HIV/AIDS Research Division of the University of KwaZulu Natal (www.heard.org.za); and program-level interventions by NGOs (Mullins 2002).

Box 8. Benefits of mainstreaming HIV/AIDS priorities into poverty-reduction strategies

- HIV/AIDS priorities become an integral part of a government's development agenda, giving the epidemic greater political visibility and leadership.
- HIV/AIDS is more likely to feature prominently in the priorities of the ministries of finance and planning, and such attention is a prerequisite for full government mobilization in the fight against HIV/AIDS and its socioeconomic impact.
- The government takes firm charge of the national AIDS program, which consequently enjoys stronger national ownership and the oversight necessary for real and sustained results.
- The response to HIV/AIDS becomes properly institutionalized and integrated into all activities of government, across all sectors, and is not the exclusive domain of the ministry of health and charity-focused NGOs. The response becomes truly multisectoral and multilevel, with better coordination between various sectors and actors and between national and local-level interventions. The result is a scaled-up and sustained nationwide response.
- Domestic resources are allocated to the national HIV/AIDS strategic plan, avoiding too much dependency on donor-driven program design and financing (while not ignoring the fact that much more donor support is required to bridge the gap between available resources and resource needs).
- Debt-relief savings are more likely to be earmarked for HIV/AIDS interventions as part of the national poverty-reduction strategy, providing an important opportunity to increase the level of public spending on HIV/AIDS. (Of the 42 countries eligible for HIPC debt relief, 30 are seriously affected by HIV/AIDS.)
- The national AIDS program can benefit from accountability frameworks developed in the context of budget planning and poverty-reduction strategies, thus producing a clear division of labor between various government institutions and transparent allocation and disbursement of resources.

Source: UNDP 2002.

Mainstreaming should be outcome- as well as input-led. It is not enough to apply an HIV lens to programs; it is also necessary to ensure that outcomes are tracked. HIV-relevant indicators need to be built into program monitoring and evaluation systems. Again, it is not necessary to reinvent food and nutrition security indicators, but the lens should be applied to existing ones. A balance has to be found between indicators that allow comparison across communities and administrative units and context-specific indicators arising from a community-driven process.

But even in countries where HIV/AIDS is deeply rooted and where the policy environment has been the most conducive to prevention and mitigation strategies, multisectoral responses appear limited. Many ministries of agriculture and major donors have yet to mainstream HIV/AIDS responses into their policy processes. Where organizations have become involved—whether agricultural agencies taking HIV/AIDS into consideration or AIDS organizations factoring in food security—the efforts have typically been made in isolation.

Box 9. Networking for action: RENEWAL in Africa

One currently active partnership is the Regional Network on HIV/AIDS, Rural Livelihoods and Food Security (RENEWAL) comprising stakeholders from Uganda, Malawi, Zambia, South Africa, and recently Kenya. Facilitated by IFPRI, RENEWAL is developing processes through which decision makers at different levels and in different contexts can learn to use the HIV/AIDS lens. These processes, which are linked, currently include (1) the formation of sector-wide national networks that advance practical understanding through action research and forums for exchange and policy dialogue; (2) the review of national agricultural policies and programs; and (3) the development of community-led action on food security and livelihoods to advance prevention, mitigation, care, and treatment.

RENEWAL is an evolving, regional network of networks. It started life in 2001 as a hub-and-spoke network, wherein national networks were in two-way communication with the IFPRI/ISNAR (International Service for National Agricultural Research) hub—essentially a North–South linkage. It is now evolving toward a spider's-web network, wherein South–South communications between different national networks and between national networks and other partners and networks are increasing in breadth and depth. The human infrastructure of RENEWAL comprises in-country national network coordinators advised by a national advisory panel, with the national networks comprising informal groupings of researchers, policymakers, program managers, NGO staff, UN representatives, and others.

RENEWAL's activities relate to its three core principles: targeted action research, capacity strengthening, and policy communications. Action research is aimed at filling the gaps in understanding of the reciprocal relationship between HIV/AIDS and food and nutrition insecurity that are currently constraining effective action. Current and planned policies and programs are analyzed in terms of their impact on prevention or mitigation, and RENEWAL supports experiments to enhance the positive effects and reduce the negative ones. More details may be found at www.ifpri.org/renewal.

Generating a truly multisectoral and mainstreamed response will require creating institutional incentives and developing the capacity for horizontal, team-oriented approaches rather than vertical, sector-led programs. Incentives are also needed to develop partnerships—between policymakers and researchers (see Box 9), between community organizations and NGOs and government, and between the public and private sectors.

Box 10. Frameworks for action

Global frameworks

Millennium Development Goals (MDGs), adopted by the UN General Assembly in September 2000

General Assembly Special Session on HIV/AIDS (UNGASS) Declaration of Commitment in June 2001, which set goals to be achieved by 2003 and 2005

Regional frameworks

Abuja Declaration on HIV/AIDS, Tuberculosis and Other Related Infectious Diseases in April 2001, endorsed by African Union member states

New Partnership for Africa's Development (NEPAD), launched July 2001 to tackle social, economic, and political priorities across the continent

Commission on HIV/AIDS and Governance in Africa (CHGA), created in 2003 in response to HIV/AIDS, subregional crises, and governance challenges, chaired by the UN Economic Commission for Africa (ECA)

Next Steps for Action in Southern Africa: A Report of the Special Envoy of the Secretary-General for Humanitarian Needs in Southern Africa, Inter-Agency Standing Committee, April 2003

UNAIDS response to the AIDS crisis in southern Africa, April 2003

Southern African Development Community (SADC) frameworks

SADC HIV/AIDS Strategic Framework and Programme of Action, 2003–7: aims to reduce infections, mitigate socioeconomic impact, develop policies and legislation, and mobilize resources

Maseru Declaration on the Fight against HIV/AIDS in the SADC Region, July 2003: reaffirms the commitment of SADC governments to urgently combat HIV/AIDS through multisectoral strategic action

National frameworks

Poverty-reduction strategy papers (PRSPs) and other national-development frameworks

National AIDS strategic plans

Source: United Nations 2004.

Coordination and collaboration are improving as the truly crosscutting nature of HIV/AIDS is at last being internalized and addressed in international and national strategies. There is growing recognition that national responses need to be grounded in strategic frameworks (see Box 10). UNAIDS has usefully proposed the "Three Ones" commitment: each country should have one HIV/AIDS strategy, one HIV/AIDS commission, and one way of measuring and reporting progress, and it is being supported in this proposal by DFID (DFID 2003b). The United Nations system has proposed a systemwide response that includes 11 priority programmatic and 11 institutional actions (United Nations 2004).

In addition to organizational scaling up at the government level, locally relevant, community-driven approaches should be expanded. Much recent research has been done by the World Bank and others on the factors determining the success of the scaling up of such programs, and many of the lessons are relevant to HIV/AIDS contexts (see Box 11).

Box 11. Scaling up community-driven development (CDD): Key lessons

- Overall, keep in mind context, institutional arrangements, capacity, and the triggers and different processes of scaling up.
- Donors and governments need to think of the process beyond the project—of transformation or transition, not exit. Need to balance push and pull factors and avoid "supply-driven demand-driven development." Community-driven is citizen-driven, not client-driven.
- Capacity is pivotal and consists of more than simply resources; because it includes motivation and commitment, appropriate incentives are necessary at all levels. Capacity development takes time and resources but is an essential investment. The capacity and commitment of facilitators and local leaders are particularly important.
- Learn by doing—and by communicating, monitoring, evaluating, and changing. Learn from failure, but learn faster from success. Start with the positive (what's working), not the problem (what isn't), and build on that. Be adaptive, flexible, and open to change. Anticipate and address trade-offs. Apply realistic time horizons (10- to 15-year, not 5-year, cycles).
- Build library of well-documented, context-specific experiences through good monitoring, evaluation, and operational research. Use these to advocate for contextually appropriate improvements.
- To sustain CDD, anchor it within existing contextual systems (government), frameworks (such as PRSP), and processes (decentralization), even where these may be imperfect. The ultimate aim is to weave and embed sustainable CDD into the national social, political, cultural, and institutional fabric.

Source: Gillespie 2004.

Chapter 6

Conclusions

Prevention, care, treatment, and mitigation should remain the building blocks of a comprehensive approach to combating HIV/AIDS. To the extent that they are exacerbated by AIDS, food and nutrition insecurity will also be reduced through such efforts. But these fundamental approaches should not be compartmentalized. Together they represent a continuum or web of mutually reinforcing responses. Mitigation, for example, can be preventive if it succeeds in dealing with risks generated by people being, or becoming, food-insecure. Care is also preventive: programs aimed at improving the physical, economic, social, and spiritual well-being of people with HIV may reduce transmission risk. Orphans who are cared for by the extended family or community are less likely to engage in risky sexual practices than if they are left to fend for themselves on the street. And treatment is also preventive: as viral load is reduced, so is infectivity. Each one of these elements is necessary, but insufficient in itself, in the overall war response to HIV/AIDS.

Food and nutrition security are fundamentally important to the prevention, care, treatment, and mitigation of HIV/AIDS. Food insecurity and malnutrition raise risks of HIV exposure and infection. A program of care without a nutritional component is like a leaky bucket; the efficacy of antiretroviral drug treatment may be compromised by malnutrition, and any mitigation strategy must take account of the fact that what those affected need most is usually food, at a time when their ability to acquire food may be diminished.

Although our knowledge of these interactions has grown enormously over the last few years, gaps remain (see Loevinsohn and Gillespie 2003a). We need to understand better how agricultural and other livelihood systems, policy, and practice—in urban as well as rural areas—contribute to the spread of HIV. We need more longitudinal studies that capture the local dynamics of impact and response in different situations, particularly among households and communities who are actively strengthening their own resistance and resilience through innovative responses. The contextual specificity of key interactions is insufficiently recognized, as witnessed by the frequent, heroic extrapolation of observations from cross-sectional studies into universally representative "facts." And, finally, we need to build the evidence base on action. Indicators and monitoring systems need to be put in place to track the effectiveness of policies and programs aimed at responding to the interaction of HIV/AIDS with food and nutrition insecurity.

To come to grips with these challenges and effectively fill our knowledge gaps, we need to build bridges between social scientists, epidemiologists, public-health specialists, nutritionists, and agricultural economists. Only thus will the causes and consequences of HIV/AIDS be mapped in ways that facilitate effective action. The key concepts of resistance and resilience, for example, straddle various disciplines, from the biology of immune function to the sociology of community cohesion, and progress can be made as light is shone on these interfaces. Community resilience depends to some degree on individual resilience, which is manifested in part by nutritional well-being. The converse is also true: resilient community institutions can provide the space and opportunity for people to secure their livelihoods and provision themselves with adequate food and nutrition.

Although there is growing appreciation of the fact that AIDS is a major problem for development, not just health, we do not, as some might argue, need a whole battery of new AIDS programs. Such a view is not only inaccurate but also dangerous, because it adds to the prevailing sense of hopelessness. Instead, different actors, from individual household members to national policymakers, need tools and processes to turn our growing knowledge into appropriate action.

The HIV/AIDS lens is one such tool, which can be put to use in re-viewing situations and rethinking existing interventions. Programs needs to be implementable in the context of declining capacity. By mainstreaming HIV/AIDS into food and nutrition policy, we can accumulate evidence of what works under what conditions, enhance learning, and help people become better equipped to address the multiple threats of the pandemic.

Annex 1: HIV/AIDS and Food Security Evidence Base

Impact of HIV/AIDS on household size and composition

Focus of the study	Author and date	Study design	Key findings and recommendations
Household structure and factors affecting the change in household consumption among households with and without an adult death in Chiangmai Province, Thailand	Janjaroen 1998	Cross-sectional comparison of 324 households with AIDS death, non-AIDS death, and no death	Households that experienced an adult death were almost a full individual smaller than they had been prior to the death. Deaths preceded by long illness or AIDS were associated with a larger decrease in consumption than were deaths from other causes. Deaths of adult women had a stronger negative impact on consumption than deaths of adult men. Education of the household head had a protective effect on consumption of households with adult death.
The study examines the impact of an adult death on household composition, size, and economic status in Rakai district, Uganda	Menon et al. 1998	Longitudinal study of 1,945 households enrolled in a sero-prevalence study since 1989–90 and followed until 1992. Households with AIDS death, non-AIDS death, and no death were compared.	Nearly 99 percent of households with adult death vs. 45.6 percent of households with no adult death became smaller during the study. Increased dependency ratio was observed only in households with the death of an HIV-positive adult. The percent of households with no adult (15–50 years) increased nine-fold in households that experienced an adult death and twelvefold in cases where the death was of an HIV-positive adult. Decline in household durable goods occurred only in households with HIV-related death. This effect was more pronounced in agricultural than trading villages.
Impact of the AIDS epidemic on mortality and household mobility in Mwanza region, Tanzania	Urassa et al. 2001	Two sero-epidemiological surveys and ten rounds of demographic surveillance during 1994–98, with detailed interviews of households with adult death	HIV/AIDS was associated with nearly half the deaths between ages 15 and 44 years. Mortality rate of children under two years of age born to HIV-positive mothers was 2.5 times higher than children of HIV-negative mothers. In 44 percent of households in which the head died, all members moved out of the household.

Impact of young adult deaths on household dissolution, composition, migration, and coresidency arrangements of household members	Hosegood, Herbst, and Timæus 2003*	Africa Center Demographic Information System longitudinal data collected every four months in 2000 and 2001 from 10,490 households. Multivariate hazard models were used to analyze the impact of adult deaths on household structure.	Household instability was significantly associated with younger heads, female heads, and death of a household member. Five percent of households experienced at least one AIDS death during the period of observation. These households were nearly three times more likely to dissolve than other households. Child-headed households were found to be rare. Household size decreased due to both the death of a household member and outmigration of surviving members.
Impact of HIV/AIDS on household structure in Malawi	Floyd et al. 2003	Retrospective cohort study. From population-based surveys in the 1980s, 197 individuals aged 14 to 68 identified as HIV-positive were selected. A comparison group of 396 matched HIV-negative individuals was also selected. They were sought for follow-up interviews in 1998–2000.	Under-five child mortality rates were 46 percent for children born to HIV-positive mothers and 16 percent for those born to HIV-negative mothers. Only one in five marriages in which one partner was HIV-positive at the time of the baseline survey was still intact at the follow-up. Rates of remarriage of widows or divorced female spouses were lower for wives of HIV-positive men. Remarriage rates for men did not seem to be affected by the HIV status of their wives at the time of the baseline survey.
Survey in Uganda of a large sample of widows and widowers and their circumstances with regard to children, remarriage, and movement	Ntozi 1997	Data were collected in a 1992–93 survey conducted in six districts of Uganda. By a combination of purposive and random methods, 1,797 households that had experienced death since they were formed were selected as a sample.	Nearly half the spousal deaths were due to AIDS. The proportion of females widowed at the time of the study was much higher than that of males for all the six districts of the study. This is because there is a higher rate of remarriage of widowers (65.1 percent) than of widows (27.3 percent). Thirty-seven percent of widows and 17 percent of widowers migrated from their original homes. Younger spouses and those in worse health were more likely to leave. Women were more likely to leave because they are generally not entitled to inherit the land, and their kin are likely to live elsewhere.

*It is not clear whether these studies are peer-reviewed. They include research reports by organizations (e.g., Shah et al. 2001; FASAZ/FAO 2003; NAADS 2003; Parker et al. 2001), conference proceedings (e.g., Hosegood, Herbst, and Timaeus 2003; Booysen and Bachmann 2002; Mutangadura 2000; Connolly 2003; HSRC 2003), and working papers (e.g., Mather et al. 2004a; Donovan et al. 2003; Mason et al. 2003). These studies are included in the review because they are generally of high quality and have been influential in furthering the understanding of the interactions between HIV/AIDS and food and nutrition security.

Impact of HIV/AIDS on agriculture

Subsistence agriculture

Focus of the study	Author and date	Study design	Key findings and recommendations
Potential impact of AIDS on farming systems in Rwanda	Gillespie 1989	In a time- and labor-allocation analysis, the projected AIDS mortality rates of different age and sex groups, based on epidemiological models, were related to the different levels, type, and timing of their respective labor inputs in each type of farming system. Five farming systems within Rwanda were subsequently ranked with respect to their relative sensitivity to the labor loss from AIDS mortality.	Farming systems that exhibit high seasonality of labor inputs, a high degree of specialization by age and sex, a high degree of interdependence of labor inputs, increasing returns to scale of labor, and low substitutability of labor for capital are particularly vulnerable to HIV/AIDS. The farming systems were ranked as follows in order of decreasing vulnerability to AIDS-related labor loss: volcanic highlands, central Congo/Nile divide, Kivu lakeshore, high plateau, and Kagera piedmont.
Effects of HIV/AIDS on agricultural production systems and rural livelihoods in central Malawi	Shah et al. 2001*	Cross-sectional descriptive study carried out in 15 villages across three districts in central Malawi. Methodology included focus-group discussions followed by semistructured interviews with a random sample of 310 households.	Over 70 percent of the households affected by chronic sickness experienced a loss of labor. Affected households reported delayed agricultural operations (45 percent), leaving land fallow (23 percent), changes in the crop mix (26 percent), and changes in source of livelihood (36 percent). The timing and duration of the sickness (pre- or postharvest), multiple stresses, and relative economic status of the household were found to be the most critical factors determining the intensity of the impact. Women in patrilocal villages were reported to be more vulnerable to the impacts than women from matrilocal villages. Kinship networks were found to be the main source of support.

Effects of prime-age adult mortality on the time allocation of surviving household members and portfolio of farming activities	Beegle 2003	The Kagera Health and Development Survey (KHDS) surveyed over 800 households in the Kagera region up to four times from 1991 to 1994, with an average interval between surveys of 6 to 7 months.	Analysis of farm and chore hours across demographic groups found small and insignificant changes in the labor supply of individuals in households experiencing a prime-age adult death. Although some farm activities were temporarily scaled back and wage employment fell after a male death, households did not shift cultivation toward subsistence food farming and did not appear to have reduced their diversification of income sources for more than six months after the death.
A conceptual framework for analyzing the impact of AIDS on income per person at the household level	Brown, Webb, and Haddad 1994	The framework decomposes income per household member into household endowments of labor, labor-force participation, labor diversification, average supply of labor, and labor productivity. The effect on each of these of HIV/AIDS is described.	AIDS will undermine household food security. A short-sighted approach to the pandemic as simply another health problem would be a mistake. Implications for continent-wide food security are potentially huge.
Effect of working-age adult mortality on rural household size and composition, crop production, asset levels, and off-farm income in Kenya	Yamano and Jayne 2004	Two-year panel of 1,422 Kenyan households surveyed in 1997 and 2000	Household size declined by 0.64 persons among households with adult death compared to the control group, indicating partial replenishment. Larger reduction in household size due to female death than to male death was observed. No change was found in total area cropped between households incurring and not incurring an adult death. Households incurring a male adult death reduced land devoted to high-value-added crops. Those incurring the death of a female spouse/head decreased the size of cultivated area devoted to cereals. The death of household heads and spouses adversely affected the value of total crop output and value of total output per acre. Male adult death adversely affected off-farm income. Household's initial asset base seemed to exacerbate the

(continued)

Impact of HIV/AIDS on agriculture—Continued

Subsistence agriculture

Focus of the study	Author and date	Study design	Key findings and recommendations
			impact of male adult mortality only: that is, significant reductions in crop production, value of small animals, and off-farm income were observed with mortality of the male head of the household in poor families. The impacts did not decay over the three-year survey interval.
Impact of AIDS on Kagabiro village economy in Tanzania	Tibaijuka 1997	Reconnaissance survey of 220 households regarding death of adult members since 1980. Ten households with AIDS death were studied in depth.	Significant impact on agricultural production due to labor loss, reallocation of labor to nurse the ill, and disposition of assets and working capital to pay mounting medical bills were observed. Declining consumption and unsatisfactory care of orphans and elderly were also reported.
Effects of HIV/AIDS on rural communities in east and southern Africa; implications of such impacts for development in Uganda, Tanzania, and Zambia; policy implications of these findings	Barnett et al. 1995	The study was carried out in 1993, using qualitative methods in (1) three communities in Uganda, each of which was in a different stage of impact and each of which operates on a different farming system; (2) six different farming systems in Tanzania; (3) two communities with two different livelihood and farming systems in Zambia; (4) the estate sector in Zambia. The study also included detailed mapping of the vulnerability to labor loss of farming systems in Zambia.	Results showed different impacts between and within the countries. In Uganda, rural communities followed a trajectory of regressive decline in content of their production portfolio, which was more pronounced in the poorer households. In Tanzania, the study did not show any epidemic-related impacts on livelihoods, probably because the most severely affected communities were also the most food-secure. In Zambia, the farming systems most vulnerable to labor loss were not those that were most vulnerable to the epidemic. Matrilineal systems were more vulnerable to labor loss than patrilineal systems because of the instability of these households. In Tanzania, use of oxen in farming may have limited the loss of agricultural productivity, in contrast to Uganda, where oxen are not used. Authors present a generalized response strategy and detailed recommendations for action.

Impact of HIV/AIDS on land issues in Kenya, Lesotho, and South Africa	Drimie 2003	Literature review, interviews with officials, PRA methods, and semi-structured interviews with affected families	The epidemic diverted household labor and extended family away from other productive and reproductive activities as family members took care of the sick, leading to under- or nonutilization of land. The most common responses included livestock sale, hiring casual labor, lending livestock, and sharecropping. Renting was relatively uncommon because rental markets were not developed. Affected households expressed concern about their ability to negotiate fair sharecropping arrangements. These households fell below the social and economic threshold of vulnerability and "survivability," leaving survivors with limited resources having to quickly regain a sustainable livelihood. These findings indicate the importance of effective land administration systems and of land rights as HIV/AIDS affects the terms and conditions on which households and individuals hold, use, and trade land.
Specific effects felt by households when a member is ill or dies, and strategies that households develop to deal with the shocks and stress, particularly for agricultural production in Rwanda	Donovan et al. 2003*	Survey of 1,520 households in 2002. Comparisons between households with death related to illness, death unrelated to illness, and no death	Following a death, households were able to maintain their labor supply through the addition of new members. Dependency ratios were 1.6 and 2.1 for households with male and female illness respectively, above the overall average of 1.2. Reduced farm labor was reported by 60 to 80 percent of households that suffered illness or death due to illness. When a man died of illness, households cultivated less land. When a woman died or was ill, they were more likely to adopt labor-based strategies such as sharing or hiring labor. Adverse changes in diet were reported by about one-half of the households with death or illness. No strong impacts of adult death on crop production were observed. About 44 percent increases in cassava production and 120 percent increases in sweet

(continued)

Impact of HIV/AIDS on agriculture—Continued

Subsistence agriculture

Focus of the study	Author and date	Study design	Key findings and recommendations
			potato production were reported by households when a man was ill or died of illness. Households with death of a female adult saw a decline in the production of these crops. Households with an ill adult saw an increase in area planted in bananas.
Impacts of HIV/AIDS on household structures, educational status, health and health care, labor availability and gender roles, agricultural production and productivity, income-generating capacity, asset ownership, and food and nutrition security in rural Zambia	FASAZ (Farming Systems Association of Zambia)/FAO 2003*	Cross-sectional survey of 770 households (68 percent male-headed and 32 percent female-headed). Both quantitative household questionnaires and focus-group discussions were used to collect data. Households containing orphans and foster children were classified as "burdened" and compared with "unburdened" households without orphans.	Female-headed households were supporting nearly half of the orphans. Burdened households had an average of about 1.7 more members than unburdened ones and had lower per capita incomes. About 60 percent of respondents indicated that soil fertility had declined, and greater exploitation of fuel wood for sale and wild foods for home consumption were resulting in increased deforestation and the increased scarcity of wild foods. At the community level, adult malnutrition was rife, particularly in female-headed households. Almost 50 percent of the population were under 15 years of age; only 30 percent were in the productive 15–49 age group. Formal credit and savings schemes declined following the collapse of state-sponsored agricultural lending institutions. Increased involvement of children in agricultural activities, labor exchange with neighbors and relatives, shifts to less labor-demanding monocropping, reduced cropped areas, labor hiring for payment in kind, longer working days,

			and the use of minimum-tillage techniques were reported. Attempts to make up for lost income included distress sales of household assets and livestock, increased dependency on natural resources for food and income, and the establishment of clubs for group income generation.
Impacts of HIV/AIDS on individuals, households, and communities in the mixed agriculture, fisheries, and pastoral subsectors in the Lake Victoria Crescent agricultural and ecological zone	NAADS (National Agricultural Advisory Services) 2003*	A cross-sectional survey of 631 smallholder agricultural rural households at six sites. Both qualitative and quantitative data, including five-year recalls, were collected.	Agricultural and fisheries production, but not pastoral production, were reported to have decreased because of AIDS. Main household impacts included the sale of assets; reduced quality and quantity of food consumed; reductions in herd size or in the area of land cropped; reduction of crop varieties; abandonment of specific activities and crops; and removal, or stripping, of assets by relatives from outside the household. HIV/AIDS-affected households find it difficult to adopt recommended agronomic practices that boost production and the quality of produce and have less money to invest in farm inputs and implements. The dissemination of new techniques is also hampered by affected households' difficulties in attending extension seminars, their short-term planning horizons, and the death of knowledgeable extension staff. As a result of the pandemic, several institutions have emerged (such as agencies providing HIV/AIDS counseling and nutrition education), while others have collapsed (including previously established mutual-assistance networks, such as those between fish traders and fishmongers). Coping strategies were found to be erosive.

Livestock and fishing

Focus of the study	Author and date	Study design	Key findings and recommendations
Impact of HIV/AIDS on the livestock sector in two northern provinces of Namibia with the highest HIV prevalence rates	Engh et al. 2000	Review of literature and data collected through structured interviews with 24 representative farmer extension development groups and members of 22 households affected by HIV/AIDS-related sickness or death	Attending funerals and observing mourning periods resulted in an estimated loss of 25 percent of production time. Women in matrilineal families lost cattle and small livestock after the husband's death, whereas the wife's death caused no disruption. When children inherited livestock, they were found to have inadequate skills in farming and livestock management. Widespread sale and slaughter of livestock to support the sick and to provide food for the funeral mourners were found to jeopardize the livestock sector as well as crop production. About a 10 percent reduction in agriculture extension service time was reported due to the disease.
Impact of HIV/AIDS on livestock sector in Rakai, Uganda	Haslwimmer 1994	Qualitative study	Those affected by the pandemic tend to sell their large livestock and concentrate on smaller animals, such as chicken and pigs, which are often sold for cash. After the death of an adult male, widows and children are left to take care of the livestock. But they often lack the management skills to do so effectively, further eroding this asset. A 25–50 percent reduction in agriculture extension service time was reported due to the disease. HIV/AIDS was found to make farmers more receptive to innovations and more willing to organize themselves in groups.
Dynamics of inland small-scale fishing communities' livelihoods and their contexts of vulnerability at four fish-landing sites in Uganda, two on Lake Victoria (central and eastern regions) and two on Lake George (western region)	Bishop-Sambrook and Tanzarn 2003*	Data were collected through community meetings; focus-group discussions with fishing crews, boat owners, fishmongers, women, and youths; and key-informant interviews.	Three main risk factors make fishing communities highly susceptible to HIV infections: neglect by government and the service sector, a high degree of mobility, and a lack of social cohesion, reflecting the diverse and sometimes transitory nature of many fishing communities. The cash-based economy, lack of a culture of saving, and significant free time during the day also have been found to increase

high-risk behaviors. Among the most immediately vulnerable are those whose livelihood depends on their physical well-being, such as fishing crews and fish traders who cycle considerable distances to market. Although rich boat owners are at risk from HIV infection, they were the only group considered by the community to have some resilience to the impacts, derived from their relative wealth and the diversified nature of their work (hiring crew for fishing and operating small businesses). All four sites were characterized by an absence of any community initiatives to offer comfort, support, home-based care, or care for orphans. In addition, a narrow livelihood base (highly dependent on fishing) and lack of savings make the communities highly vulnerable to the impact of AIDS. Many of the sick return to their original homes, and the fishing communities were noticeably devoid of either the elderly caring for orphaned grandchildren or households fostering orphans of relatives. The authors present a susceptibility and vulnerability matrix that demonstrates the highly differentiated impacts of HIV/AIDS on fishing communities by occupation (which is often closely associated with age and sex).

The authors present four recommendations in four areas: (1) mainstreaming HIV/AIDS and the fisheries perspective into the policy agenda; (2) raising awareness of key stakeholders; (3) starting to address HIV/AIDS at the community level; and (4) promoting collaboration among various organizations to target fishing communities.

Commercial agriculture and the commercial sector

Focus of the study	Author and date	Study design	Key findings and recommendations
Direct and indirect costs of illness to firms in Zambia	Guinness et al. 2003	108 employers and employees in seven firms were interviewed to assess direct and indirect costs of illness.	The main causes of ill-health were those most frequently associated with HIV: tuberculosis (46.8 percent), diarrhea (12.9 percent), and sexually transmitted diseases (5.8 percent). Annual treatment costs to the firms ranged from Zambia kwacha (K) 60,000 to 405,000 per person treated. Other firm costs included productivity losses because of ill-health, paid sick leave, the cost of employee replacement, and funerals. Employees incurred K67,773 on average per episode of illness.
Economic impact of HIV infection in a cohort of rural sugar-mill workers in KwaZulu Natal, South Africa, from the perspective of industry	Morris et al. 2000	97 employees who tested HIV-positive between 1991 and 1998 and a control group of 100 workers who did not test positive were included in the study. Retrospective data on morbidity and mortality, including absence from work, were extracted from clinic, hospital, insurance, and employment records. These data were fed into a model projecting seroprevalence over six years.	Overall, more than a quarter of those tested, predominantly unskilled or semiskilled laborers, were HIV-positive. Over the study period 5 percent of the workforce died, and 5.7 percent retired for medical reasons. Only 58 percent of those with identified HIV infections were still active in the workforce at the end of the study, showing significant costs to the employer in terms of replacement worker costs, lost wages, and productivity losses. The authors project at least a tenfold rise in these costs over the next six years, as the current epidemic matures and HIV-infected workers develop AIDS.
The relationship between excess morbidity and mortality due to HIV and the viability of commercial agricultural sectors of Kenya	Rugalema et al. 1999*	A detailed analysis of costs incurred by six agricultural estates as a result of HIV/AIDS and firm-level coping strategies	Between 1989 and 1995, medical expenditures of the companies due to HIV/AIDS increased by US$1.15 million. Illness and death were the main reasons for employee exit from companies surveyed. Motivation and productivity of the workforce were negatively affected. Firm-level coping strategies are found to be ad hoc and reactive rather than proactive. Authors recommend formulation of workplace prevention programs.

Impact of HIV/AIDS on individual labor productivity during disease progression among workers on tea estates in western Kenya	Fox et al. 2004	Retrospective cohort design to study the productivity and attendance of 54 workers who died or were medically retired because of AIDS-related illness between 1997 and 2002. Using longitudinal regression, the workers' daily output (in kilograms of tea leaves plucked), use of paid and unpaid leave, and necessity of assignment to less strenuous tasks were compared to those of comparison workers.	HIV-positive workers plucked less tea in the 18 months preceding AIDS-related termination and used more leave in the three years before termination. After adjusting for age and environmental factors, data show that those with AIDS plucked 4.11 to 7.93 kg/day less in the last 18 months before termination than the comparison group. They used 9.2 to 11.0 more sick-leave days, 6.4 to 8.3 more annual-leave days, and 11.8 to 19.9 more casual-leave days, and they spent 19.2 to 21.8 more days doing less strenuous tasks in the two years before termination than did comparison pluckers. Tea pluckers who were terminated because of AIDS-related causes earned 16.0 percent less in their penultimate year and 17.7 percent less in the year before termination.
This study attempts to determine the impact of HIV/AIDS on agriculture and the private sector, obtain vital information on vulnerability of agriculture and the private sector to HIV/AIDS related morbidity and mortality; and identify strategies that can be implemented to prevent and control the epidemic.	Muwanga 2002*	Quantitative and qualitative survey of households in subsistence farming: 120 private commercial farms, 10 national and Swazi farms, 16 cooperative societies, and 92 businesses	HIV/AIDS has not affected the profitability and productivity of Swazi businesses, as the costs have been passed onto households and the public sector. Within the subsistence sector, family incomes have declined because of higher adult morbidity and mortality and additional expenditures on health. This decline has led to decreased food security. The response by Swazi business to the epidemic has focused mainly on avoidance of costs associated with the epidemic; absence of community investment by business and provision of limited benefits to employees leaves it to the households and public services to cater for their sick and those orphaned by the epidemic. The paper recommends that through the Ministry of Agriculture and Co-operatives, government should establish a multi-sectoral approach that goes beyond the health-based response.

(continued)

Commercial agriculture and the commercial sector—Continued

Focus of the study	Author and date	Study design	Key findings and recommendations
How South African companies minimize their AIDS-related costs by altering their benefits policies, contracts structures, and hiring practices	Rosen and Simon 2002*	Review	The authors document the systematic shifting of the AIDS-related cost burden away from the private sector to households and government. Common practices include preemployment screening, reduced employee benefits, restructured employment contracts, outsourcing of less skilled jobs, selective retrenchments, and changes in production technologies. In South Africa, more than two-thirds of large employers have reduced health-care benefits or required larger contributions by employees. Most firms have replaced defined-benefit retirement funds, which expose the firm to large annual costs but provide long-term support to families, with defined-contribution funds, which eliminate risk to the firm but provide little to families of younger workers who die of AIDS. Outsourcing of previously permanent jobs also shields firms from costs while leaving households and government to care for affected workers and their families. Many of these changes are responses to globalization and would have occurred even in the absence of AIDS, but they are devastating for employees with HIV/AIDS. Shifting the economic burden of AIDS is a predictable response by business to which a thoughtful public-policy response is needed. If a socially desirable allocation is to be achieved, countries should make explicit decisions about each sector's responsibilities.

Agricultural extension

Focus of the study	Author and date	Study design	Key findings and recommendations
The significance of HIV/AIDS for ministries of agriculture (MoAs) in eastern and southern Africa, particularly among smallholders	Topouzis 2003. See also Bota, Malindi, and Nyekanyeka 1998; GTZ 1999*	Review. Four areas of HIV/AIDS impact were analyzed in detail: (1) vulnerability of MoAs to HIV infection and the impact of AIDS; (2) disruption of MoA operations and erosion of capacity to respond to challenges posed by the HIV epidemic; (3) increased vulnerability of MoA clients to food and livelihood insecurity; (4) relevance of certain MoA policies, strategies, and programs in view of the conditions being created by HIV/AIDS.	The illness and death of people working for ministries and rural institutions are eroding the capacity of governments to respond adequately to the epidemic. Underestimation of the impact of HIV/AIDS makes it increasingly difficult for MoAs to deliver services and to cope with the crisis. MoAs and rural institutions should urgently address the implications of HIV/AIDS for their core policies and programs. The needs of a growing number of elderly people, women, and children in rural areas assuming tasks previously performed by young adult men will have to be taken into account. A client-based rather than a production-based approach is recommended. HIV/AIDS should be featured in MoAs' budgets. Identification of HIV/AIDS focal points with "soft" units can make mainstreaming of HIV/AIDS more difficult in the core areas of MoA work. Creating capacity for MoA response to HIV/AIDS requires a two-pronged approach: (1) addressing the impact of HIV/AIDS within MoAs; and (2) adjusting agricultural policies, programs, and operations to the adverse conditions created by the epidemic. Selected examples of MoA responses are reviewed and additional ways of creating capacity proposed.

(continued)

Agricultural extension—Continued

Focus of the study	Author and date	Study design	Key findings and recommendations
Extension needs of the emerging farming population and the validity of the present agricultural extension policy and programs with respect to these needs; impact of HIV/AIDS on these needs and approaches	Alleyne et al. 2001*	Nine districts from four provinces of Zambia were sampled. Study instruments included structured questionnaires (of 155 extension workers), focus-group discussions, case studies of affected households, a review of literature, and field observations.	Extension workers underestimated the level of farmers' knowledge about HIV/AIDS. Although about 55 percent of the extension workers said they discussed HIV/AIDS with their clients, the farmers reported that extension workers rarely discussed the subject with them. About 67 percent of the extension workers assessed their risk of infection as very high. About 67 percent of the respondents reported having lost a fellow worker in the last three years. The majority of agents interviewed reported a decrease in area and types of crops cultivated, increased expenditure on sickness and funerals, reduced care for crops and livestock, reduced yields, more female- and child-headed households, loss of agricultural knowledge, and reduced field labor. Attending funerals and caring for the sick were cited by 66 percent of the extension staff as the main sources of disruption of routine work. Suggestions obtained from the focus-group discussions and recommendations are presented.

Other food and nutrition-relevant impacts

Focus of the study	Author and date	Study design	Key findings and recommendations
Social and economic impacts, current and future, of HIV/AIDS on households and farming systems in Uganda; coping strategies of afflicted and affected individuals and families; effects of forced migration and refugees on the spread of HIV	Barnett and Blaikie 1992	Multiple methodologies, including approaches from epidemiology, sociology, and anthropology	Gender, age, socioeconomic status, and occupation affect rates of infection and mortality. A heuristic model illustrates the role of AIDS in changing patterns of access to resources for earning and living. Historical and contemporary data show how an interlocked set of economics and political processes led to the development of high-risk foci in which AIDS could manifest itself as it did in Buganda and Rakai districts. Coping mechanism of AIDS-affected households include diversion of healthy labor to tend to the sick, diversion of cash to medical expenses, and altered patterns of production and consumption. Recommendations for action are presented.
Changes in household expenditures and consumption due to illness and death of a household member from HIV/AIDS in Côte d'Ivoire	Bechu 1998	One hundred and seven households with at least one adult ill with AIDS and one or more children were interviewed six times at two-month intervals. The data were compared with the results of a study conducted in Yopougon in May 1992 that was based on a sample of 2,064 households.	Consumption among the AIDS-affected households was only half that of the comparison group representative of the general population. The proportion of the budget spent on health care in AIDS-affected households was almost double that of households in Yopougon. Although a slight increase in consumption was observed after the initial shock of death, the AIDS-affected households did not return to earlier levels of consumption. Health costs for the sick in the AIDS-affected households accounted for almost 80 percent of the health budget. But once the illness was identified and there was access to health care, most of the sick seemed to distance themselves gradually from the structures of modern care—and, to a lesser extent, from traditional medicine—by cutting back on hospitalization, medical consultations, and medicine.

(continued)

Other food and nutrition-relevant impacts—Continued

Focus of the study	Author and date	Study design	Key findings and recommendations
Impact of HIV/AIDS on individuals and households in Free State, South Africa	Booysen and Bachmann 2002*	A cross-sectional comparison of households affected and not affected by HIV/AIDS in two communities of Free State: Welkom (urban) and QwaQwa (rural). HIV-affected households were those in which at least one person was known to be HIV-positive.	Household members, mainly those who were unemployed, spent an average of 7.5 hrs per day providing care during the fatal illness of the deceased. Per capita adult equivalent income in affected households was only between 50 and 60 percent of the levels of income in nonaffected households. The average monthly food expenditure of affected households was 70 to 80 percent of that in nonaffected households, although no significant difference was found in total monthly expenditures. Households with access to medical aid were least likely to resort to using up financial savings.
Impacts on households of female mortality in Zimbabwe; household coping mechanisms and formal and informal social-support mechanisms	Mutangadura 2000	A descriptive analysis of a sample of 215 households fostering maternal orphans	Major household impacts include food insecurity, decrease in school attendance, increased work burden on children, and loss of assets. Elderly women became the leading foster parents of surviving maternal orphans. Households are dependent on informal sources of support to help cushion the impacts of premature adult female mortality.
Economic impact of HIV/AIDS on rural households in Limpopo Province, South Africa	Oni et al. 2002	Cross-sectional data obtained from 680 rural households	HIV/AIDS-affected households had lower annual income, were smaller in size, had lower savings, and spent more on transportation, funerals, and health care, but less on housing, remittances, and education than unaffected households. The coping strategies adopted by affected households included sale of household assets, withdrawal of children from schools, and joining community support groups.

Response of households to prime-age mortality; strategies used by households to respond to illness and death; implications for design of agricultural polices and programs in Mozambique	Mather et al. 2004a*	Nationally representative household panel survey from 1999 and 2002. Afflicted households were defined as those that suffered illness or death in the last four years.	Cash, livestock, assets, and total and per-adult-equivalent income were lower for households experiencing a death. Affected households had lower total and cultivated land area, particularly following the death of a male household head. But cultivated area per adult equivalent among the households experiencing death was similar to that of non-affected households. Households with a female prime-age death were more likely to have children leaving the household and to have a new female adult arrive. A male death did not result in departure of children or an increased arrival of adult males compared with the nonaffected households. Thus, although all adult deaths resulted in household size reduction, households with a female death were better able to adjust (showing lower dependency ratios). Households with a male death were more likely to hire or share labor than households with a female death. Death of a household head increased the likelihood of use of child labor. Implications for the ministry of agriculture are discussed.
Whether HIV/AIDS increased household's likelihood of falling below poverty line in Rungwe district Tanzania	Mwakalobo 2003*	Cross-sectional survey of 119 households in three villages	Households experiencing AIDS death spent substantially less on food than those not experiencing death. Logistics regression results reveal that HIV/AIDS-related death significantly increases the probability of a household falling below the poverty line.
Economic, education, health, and nutrition outcomes for AIDS-affected families when one or both the breadwinners of the families died in Zambia	Nampanya-Serpell 2000	Five-year retrospective study of AIDS-affected families. Structured interviews were conducted in 232 urban and 101 rural, AIDS-affected families.	A decline in monthly disposable income of more than 80 percent was observed in more than two-thirds of the AIDS-affected families, especially following paternal death. Family displacement to poorer sites with fewer services in urban areas, and labor loss resulting in food insecurity in rural areas were observed. Younger children were more vulnerable to poor nutrition and ill-health than

(continued)

Other food and nutrition-relevant impacts—Continued

Focus of the study	Author and date	Study design	Key findings and recommendations
			older children. Socioeconomic status of the caregiving families (but not gender) in the urban sample was protective against dropping out of school. In the rural sample, age of the orphans (but not socioeconomic status) was found to be a predictor of educational outcomes, with older orphans more likely to drop out than younger ones.
Household responses to death, and the reasons why some households manage better than others	Lundberg and Over 2000	Panel data set from Kagera region, Tanzania	Wealthy households were wealthy not only in physical and human assets but also in social assets or social capital and were more likely to receive material aid than poorer households. Poor households instead received loans through formal credit, suggesting that the crisis is potentially worse for them, as they may be unable to repay loans on time and lose collateral. Recommendations include providing better-targeted assistance to those with few alternative sources of support.
Dubious value of the concept of coping strategies in assessing the HIV/AIDS crisis	Rugalema 2000	Conceptual	Coping strategies imply the analysis of success rather than failure. The strategies adopted by the households affected by adult mortality in fact often represent a failure to cope.
The literature on household and community coping strategies to HIV/AIDS	Mutangadura et al. 1999	Review	Affected households were seen to adopt strategies aimed at improving food security, raising and supplementing income to maintain household expenditure patterns, and

			alleviating loss of labor. Some coping strategies render households insecure and vulnerable. Communities have developed traditional and modern responses to HIV/AIDS, including labor sharing, orphan support, community-based child care, and credit schemes for funeral benefits. Community-based organizations receiving external funding have been found to be very beneficial to many affected households. Policy recommendations are included.
Effect of adult mortality and morbidity due to AIDS on livelihood of households in one village in Bukoba district, Tanzania	Rugalema 1999	Intensive, village-based case study conducted from February to December 1996.The village had 167 households, out of which 52 were afflicted (included at least one member ill with AIDS or had lost a member to AIDS) and 47 were affected by HIV/AIDS (were not directly afflicted but were diverting resources to help others, such as extended family, who were afflicted).	Labor is diverted from productive activities to provide care to the sick. AIDS-induced illness consumes cash, productive assets, and social claims, particularly the use of external labor. Funerals deplete the resources of afflicted and affected households. AIDS has induced changes in organization of funerals, cropping patterns, and agronomic and stockkeeping practices as a result of asset and labor depletion among afflicted households. Inheritance of property among survivors, especially orphans and widows, may be at issue. Survivors confront difficulties in getting access to resources.

Impacts on human capital

Focus of the study	Author and date	Study design	Key findings and recommendations
Impact of adult mortality on morbidity, height for age, and weight for height of children under five in Tanzania; efficacy of health interventions in mitigating the impact of adult mortality	Ainsworth and Semali 2000	Kagera Health and Development Survey (KHDS) panel data set	Adult death (recent adult deaths and orphanhood) had an independent effect on reported morbidity and height for age in children. The loss of parents or other adults in the household worsened height-for-age measures. The loss of a parent increased stunting among the nonpoor to levels found among poor children living with parents; among the poor, orphanhood increased stunting even further. Children in the poorest households, those with uneducated parents, and those with the least access to health care were most severely affected. Immunization against measles, oral rehydration, and access to health care disproportionately improved health outcomes among the poorest children, and within that group among children affected by adult mortality.
Effect of accommodating an orphan on household welfare; likelihood of foster children having reduced access to public services in Uganda	Deininger, Garcia, and Subbarao 2003	Surveys conducted in 1992 and 2000. A panel of 1,300 households included in both periods was included in the analysis.	Orphans' health and nutritional status were worse than those of nonorphans. Their access to public services was found to be less than that of children who lived with their biological parents. Fostering households consumed less, saved less, and invested less, with serious implications for aggregate savings and investment in the economy. After the adoption of universal primary education, being a foster child no longer conveyed a disadvantage with respect to access to education. However, in the absence of proactive polices, access of young foster children to health services worsened over time.
Impact of parental death and disability on investments in child human capital	Gertler et al. 2003	Panel data sets from Indonesia and Mexico	The death of a prime-age adult household member resulted in reduction in consumption per capita in both countries. In Mexico no recovery was observed even after 12

			months. Bereaved children were more likely to drop out of school than nonbereaved children in both countries. In Indonesia, paternal deaths had a lower impact on school enrollment than maternal deaths; in Mexico, the reverse was true. Maternal orphans had a higher probability of dying (1.8 percent higher in Indonesia and 1.5 percent in Mexico) than nonbereaved children. Maternal death increased the probability of wasting (by 15 percent in Indonesia) but not stunting.
Evaluation of an orphan-support program in Uganda	Gilborn et al. 2001*	The baseline sample included 353 HIV-positive parents, 495 children of PLWHAs, 233 orphans, and 326 guardians. Parents or guardians, older children (aged 13–17), and orphan support program staff were interviewed, and focus group discussions were conducted.	About 66 percent of HIV-positive parents were widowed, and 40 percent indicated taking in a foster child. HIV-positive parents expressed concerns about their children's access to education and food, and lack of an appropriate guardian. About 50 percent of the adult respondents reported property-grabbing as a problem. Among older children of PLWHAs, declines in school attendance (28 percent) and school performance (26 percent) were reported. Older foster children showed improvements in school attendance (22 percent). Children of PLWHAs spent significantly more time on taking care of the sick and young children. Access to food was cited as a major problem.
Impact of AIDS on primary-school enrollment in Kenya	Yamano and Jayne forthcoming	Panel of 1,266 households surveyed in 1997, 2000, and 2002	Working-age adult mortality correlated strongly with lagged prevalence rates at nearby sentinel survey sites. Children in relatively poor households were more likely to drop out of school after the death of an adult member than children in less poor households. The lagged HIV prevalence rate correlated negatively with schooling among the poor, even after controlling for child fixed effects. Adult mortality negatively affected schooling even in the period directly before the death, possibly because children were sharing the burden of caregiving.

(continued)

Impacts on human capital—Continued

Focus of the study	Author and date	Study design	Key findings and recommendations
Prevalence of and consequences for existing child-care practices in a rural area with moderately high HIV prevalence in Tanzania	Urassa et al. 1997	Cross-sectional descriptive analysis of Kisesa community, conducted between 1994 and 1996	8.9 percent of children under 15 years of age lost one or both parents. Households with orphans did not have a lower economic status but had less favorable dependency ratios. Orphans and foster children had significantly lower school enrollment and higher dropout rates than children living with both parents. Orphan and foster children were more mobile than other children.
Impact of orphanhood on school enrollment in ten sub-Saharan African countries	Case et al. 2004	Data from 19 DHS studies conducted in ten countries between 1992 and 2000	Orphans are less likely to be in school than are nonorphans, including nonorphans with whom they live. Children who live in households headed by nonparental relatives fare systematically worse than those who live with parents, and those who live in households headed by nonrelatives fare worse still. Much of the gap between the schooling of orphans and nonorphans is explained by the tendency of orphans to live with distant relatives or unrelated caregivers.

HIV/AIDS and food crises

Focus of the study	Author and date	Study design	Key findings and recommendations
Child nutrition and the 2002–3 food crisis in Lesotho, Malawi, Mozambique, Swaziland, Zambia, and Zimbabwe	Mason et al. 2003*	Data on child nutritional status and HIV/AIDS from various sources in six countries	The 2002 drought in southern Africa interacted with HIV/AIDS in high-prevalence areas to bring about a rapid deterioration in child nutrition. However, because these effects were seen mainly in areas that previously had better child nutrition, the effect is not obvious from averages. HIV (which is more prevalent in urban areas) is leveling out the previous urban/rural nutritional differentials. Underweight increased very substantially, for example, from 5 percent to 20 percent in Maputo (Mozambique) between 1997 and 2002; from 17 percent to 32 percent in Copperbelt (Zambia) from 1999 to 2001–2; and from 11 percent to 26 percent in Midlands Province (Zimbabwe) from 1999 to 2002. Changes were much smaller during nondrought periods and in areas of lower HIV prevalence. These trends may be partly explained by direct effects of pediatric AIDS (growth failure is occurring at younger ages), but the larger effect is probably indirect, as drought and HIV hasten destitution in affected families. Traditionally worse-off areas appeared protected, perhaps because of food assistance; this impact remains to be determined. A nontraditional vulnerable group is emerging in the better-off areas, to which resources need to be directed. The causes may include poorer child care as well as food insecurity (for orphans and others). Heightened surveillance and preparation for returning drought are recommended. Monitoring for future

(continued)

HIV/AIDS and food crises—Continued

Focus of the study	Author and date	Study design	Key findings and recommendations
			deterioration should continue. New means should be identified for supporting the child population, most of whom are affected at least indirectly.
Interactions between HIV/AIDS, food insecurity, and famine during the 2002–3 food crisis in southern Africa	Harvey 2004	Review and field work; interviews with various humanitarian organizations in Malawi, Zambia, Zimbabwe, and South Africa	HIV/AIDS is one of many factors contributing to underlying vulnerability. HIV/AIDS undermines the ways in which people have traditionally coped with famine and acute crisis. It may increase mortality in famines because people with AIDS are less able to cope with reduced food intake and the additional disease burden arising from social disruption. Issues associated with crises may exacerbate the risks of transmission of HIV/AIDS and contribute to the spread of the epidemic. Lessons learned by the humanitarian community from the crisis in southern Africa are summarized, and avenues for improving field operations and management are identified.
Reasons why the 2002–3 food crisis is different from conventional drought-induced food shortages; the "new-variant famine" hypothesis	De Waal and Whiteside 2003	Conceptual	The HIV/AIDS epidemic in southern Africa may explain why many households are facing food shortage and limited recovery. Four factors are new: (1) household labor shortages are attributable to adult morbidity and mortality, as is the rise in numbers of dependents; (2) increased adult mortality causes loss of assets and skills; (3) sick adults and children orphaned by AIDS impose a heavy burden of care; and (4) vicious interactions exist between malnutrition and HIV. In so-called new-variant famine, the descent to destitution may be much more rapid, and the possibilities for recoveries are much reduced.

Contribution of HIV and AIDS to problems faced by rural households in southern Africa during the 2002 food emergency	SADC FANR 2003*	Data generated from emergency food-security assessments conducted in Malawi and Zambia in August and December 2002 and from Zimbabwe in August 2002	Households affected by adult morbidity and mortality and with a high demographic load were significantly more vulnerable to food security shocks than other households. They suffered from marked reductions in agricultural production and income, leading to earlier engagement in distress coping strategies, and, ultimately, a decline in food security. Key differences relate to whether the household had an active adult or a chronically ill person present, whether the head of household was chronically ill, the dependency ratio, and whether the household had taken in orphaned children. Each of these characteristics had further nuances that were affected by age and gender.
Livelihood strategies and the contribution of food aid to food security in the 2002–3 food crisis; linkages between HIV/AIDS and food security	Zambia VAC and SADC FANR VAC 2003*	VAC assessment data. The study compared food security outcomes among households affected by HIV/AIDS and those not affected.	Between March 2002 and April 2003, most people in Zambia met their energy requirements. For those under stress, coping strategies focused mainly on changes to food consumption rather than strategies that reduced household assets. Households affected by HIV/AIDS were more likely to cite lack of labor as a reason for limiting cultivated land than households not affected. HIV/AIDS-affected households were also more likely to report a reduction in education expenditures. However, no association was found between food production and HIV/AIDS.

Impacts of food and nutrition insecurity on spread of HIV

Focus of the study	Author and date	Study design	Key findings and recommendations
Social and economic features of the HIV/AIDS epidemic in the United Kingdom, Botswana, Uganda, India, and Ukraine	Barnett and Whiteside 1999	Review and conceptual	Certain features of the society and economy are key determinants of the degree to which epidemics become generalized. These features can be conceptualized in ways that assist in more effective targeting of preventive interventions and measures to confront the medium- and long-term effects of raised morbidity and mortality associated with the occurrence of generalized HIV/AIDS epidemics.
Susceptibility and vulnerability of a society to HIV	Barnett and Whiteside 2000	Conceptual and theoretical	Susceptibility and vulnerability are determined by two variables: the degree of social cohesion and the overall level of wealth of the society. Four broad types of societies can be distinguished, each with a distinctive epidemic pattern of HIV prevalence. Social cohesion can be strengthened in four areas: (1) altering social norms and standards; (2) improving the status of women; (3) improving the performance of social institutions; and (4) improving the quality of controlled social environments —for example, improving housing and social support for migrant-labor camps.
Factors that could explain differences in rate of spread of HIV between different regions in sub-Saharan Africa (Benin, Cameroon, Kenya, and Zambia)	Auvert et al. 2001	In each of the cities chosen (two with high and two with low HIV prevalence) in four countries, a representative sample of about 1,000 men and 1,000 women aged 15–49 years was tested for HIV. Information on behavior, socioeconomic background, and STDs was also obtained between 1997 and 1998.	High-risk sexual behavior was not more common in the cities with high HIV prevalence than in those with low prevalence, but HSV-2 infection and lack of circumcision were consistently more prevalent. The authors conclude that biological factors outweigh differences in sexual behavior in explaining the variation in rate of spread of HIV in the four cities.

The relation between malnutrition and HIV prevalence	Stillwaggon 2002	Cross-country analysis of 44 countries. The dependent variable was HIV prevalence, and the independent variables were changes in caloric and protein intake, change in urban population, Gini coefficient, and real per capita GDP between 1970 and 1995.	The greater the decrease in caloric intake and the more unequal the income distribution, the higher the rate of HIV infection. Differences in sexual behavior cannot explain vast differences in rates of HIV transmission between sub-Saharan Africa and most of the rest of the world. Models for HIV transmission for poor populations must include other variables, including host factors conventionally recognized as influencing susceptibility to infectious diseases.
Socioeconomic characteristics of adults who died from AIDS and those who died from other causes in Tanzania	Ainsworth and Semali 1998	Stratified random sample of 800 households in Kagera region, interviewed from 1991 to 1994	Those who died of AIDS were nearly 15 years younger, on average, than those who died of other causes and only slightly older than those who lived. For both men and women, the probability of dying of AIDS was highest for those who had completed primary schooling, whereas the probability of death from other causes was highest for those with no schooling or only a few years of primary education. Farmers of both sexes have the lowest probability of death from causes other than AIDS compared with other occupations; 73 percent of men and 88 percent of women were farmers in this pooled sample. There was no relation between physical assets and the probability of dying of AIDS for adults of either gender, nor for the probability of death from other causes for women.
Prevalence of HIV-1 infection and its relation to socioeconomic and obstetric history factors in rural Gutu district, Zimbabwe	Nilses et al. 2000	A cross-sectional study of women 15 to 44 years of age in 12 randomly selected villages	The multivariate logistic regression showed an increased risk of HIV infection for women aged 20 to 39 years compared with women aged 15 to 19 years, and for women who were divorced, widowed, or separated compared with those who were unmarried.
Relationships between women's empowerment and HIV prevention at national and individual levels, with a focus on Botswana	Greig and Koopman 2003	A preliminary quantitative survey of 71 sexually active women in Gaborone, Botswana, conducted in February 2001	HIV prevalence was positively correlated with indirect indicators of women's empowerment relating to their education (female enrollment in secondary education and female-to-male ratio in secondary school enrollment), but

(continued)

Impacts of food and nutrition insecurity on spread of HIV—Continued

Focus of the study	Author and date	Study design	Key findings and recommendations
			not to their economic status (as measured by proportion of women in paid employment in industry and services) or political status (proportion of women in national parliament), controlling for gross national income, percentage of births attended by health professionals, and percentage of roads paved. Condom use at last sexual encounter positively and significantly correlated with both indicators of women's educational empowerment but was not significantly related to the other two indices. Regression analyses showed that women's negotiating power and economic independence were the factors most strongly related to condom use; they did not show that education was a crucial factor. Economic independence was the factor most strongly related to negotiating power. These results suggest that in Botswana, HIV prevention efforts may need to improve women's negotiating skills and access to income-generating activities.
The effect of community characteristics on HIV prevalence and incidence	Bloom et al. 2002	Data from an open-cohort study were used to examine the association between individual and community risk factors and HIV prevalence in 1994–95 and incidence between 1994–95 and 1996–97 among men and women. Logistic and Cox regression models were used to assess community effects, controlling for multiple individual factors.	All four community factors (level of social and economic activity, ratio of bar workers to male population aged 18 to 59, level of community mobility, and distance to nearest town) had strong effects on HIV transmission. Men who lived in subvillages with the highest level of social and economic activity were about five times more likely to be HIV-positive and women about twice as likely than those in places with low levels of activity. The strong association between community characteristics and HIV incidence could not be explained by differences in individual risk factors. The association between HIV incidence and

			community factors was in the expected direction but did not reach statistical significance.
Implications of the generalized heterosexual epidemic of AIDS in Africa for Latin America	Stillwaggon 2000	Cross-country multivariate regression analysis of 20 Latin American and Caribbean countries	Statistical analysis shows the duality of the AIDS epidemic. HIV prevalence is strongly correlated with higher real GDP per capita, urbanization, labor migration, and low calorie intake.
Factors that could explain differences in the spread of HIV within sub-Saharan African populations	Boerma et al. 2003	Ecologic comparison of data from population-based surveys in rural areas of high and relatively low HIV prevalence in Zimbabwe (Manicaland) and Tanzania (Kisesa)	HIV prevalences were 15.4 percent and 5.3 percent in men aged 17 to 44 years and 21.1 percent and 8.0 percent in women aged 15 to 44 years (odds ratios, 3.3 and 3.1 respectively). In Manicaland marriage is later, spatial mobility more common, cohabitation with marital partners less frequent, education levels higher, and male circumcision less common. However, adjustments for differences in these factors increased the odds ratios for HIV infection in Manicaland compared to Kisesa to 6.9 and 4.8 for men and women respectively. Sexually transmitted infection levels were similar, but syphilis was common in Kisesa. Respondents in Kisesa started sexual activity earlier and reported more sexual partners. Age differences between partners were similar in the two locations. Substantial differences exist between the contemporary sociodemographic profiles of rural Manicaland and Kisesa. However, these differences did not translate into measurable differences in the biological or behavioral factors for which data were available and did not explain the much higher HIV prevalence in Manicaland. These findings might reflect more extensive AIDS-selective mortality and behavior change or greater bias in reporting of sexual behavior in Zimbabwe.

(continued)

Impacts of food and nutrition insecurity on spread of HIV—Continued

Focus of the study	Author and date	Study design	Key findings and recommendations
Prevalence of, and risk factors for, HIV infection among women in an urban South African setting	Zuma et al. 2003	A random sample of 834 women was recruited into a community-based, cross-sectional study	HIV prevalence was 37.1 percent, with higher prevalence among migrant women (46.0 percent) than nonmigrant women (34.7 percent) (odds ratio [OR], 1.61, 95 percent confidence interval [CI], 1.11 to 2.31). The highest HIV prevalence (50.9 percent) was among women aged 26 to 35. Having had two or more sexual partners increased the risk of HIV infection (OR, 4.88; 95 percent CI, 3.01 to 7.89). Migration, age, marital status, alcohol use, syphilis, and gonorrhea were independently associated with HIV infection. Recommendations include provision of services to treat STDs and educational empowerment programs to promote safer sex among migrant women.
The relationship between population mobility and multipartner sex and their implications for the spread of HIV and AIDS in Botswana	Hope 2001	Structured and unstructured interviews with a sample of 292 mobile workers in rural and urban settings in four selected districts of the country. Focus-group discussions were conducted at all sites.	Men dominate the mobile-worker sector in Botswana. About 56 percent of all mobile workers were single; 5 percent of women mobile workers were single. A majority of workers had a live-in partner at the location of their employment. Of these workers, 44 percent had some level of secondary education, 38 percent had attended or completed primary schooling. Thirty-seven percent visited home monthly, and 23 percent visited every weekend. Fifty-three percent of the mobile workers had sexual intercourse 2 to 5 times per week. Forty-nine percent never used condoms. Ninety-seven percent were aware of the disease. About 33 percent of those interviewed said they were aware of a fellow worker who had contracted HIV/AIDS. One-quarter of them indicated having a family member who had contracted or died of HIV/AIDS.

The relationship between behavior and the epidemic in Swaziland	Whiteside et al. 2003*	Literature review and workshops	HIV prevalence rates in Swaziland, unlike those elsewhere, seem to vary little between rural and urban areas and districts. HIV prevalence may be reaching a plateau but in all likelihood will rise by a few more percentage points. Because Swaziland's population is youthful, the epidemic will have an inbuilt momentum. The apparent high level of sexually transmitted infections will increase the spread of HIV. Although the level of knowledge regarding HIV is generally good, people feel that they do not know enough. Youths attending school have low levels of sexual activity (70 percent are not sexually active); the converse is true for those not in school (more than 70 percent are sexually active). The social drivers of HIV/AIDS include culture and women's status, along with poverty, inequality, and mobility.
Epidemiology of HIV infection in rural West Africa	Lagarde et al. 2003	A comparative cross-sectional study using a standardized questionnaire and biological tests was conducted in three communities with contrasting infection levels: two rural communities in Senegal (Niakhar and Bandafassi, 866 and 952 adults, respectively) and one in Guinea-Bissau (Caio, 1,416 adults). The investigators compared the distribution of population characteristics and analyzed individuals' risk factors for HIV infection in Caio.	The level of HIV infection was very low in Niakhar (0.3 percent) and Bandafassi (0.0 percent), but 10.5 among adults in Caio, mostly HIV-2. Mobility was prevalent at all the sites. Short-term mobility was found to be a risk factor for HIV infection among men in Caio (adjusted odds ratio [aOR], 2.06; 95 percent CI, 1.06 to 3.99). Women from Caio who reported casual sex in a city during the past 12 months were much more likely to be infected with HIV (OR, 5.61; 95 percent CI, 1.56 to 20.15). Short-term mobility was associated with risk behaviors at all sites.

(continued)

Impacts of food and nutrition insecurity on spread of HIV—Continued

Focus of the study	Author and date	Study design	Key findings and recommendations
Influence of relative socioeconomic status on the sexual behaviors of women and men aged 14 to 24 years in KwaZulu Natal Province, South Africa, an environment characterized by high HIV prevalence and high rates of poverty and inequality	Hallman 2004	Household survey data collected in 2001	Relative economic disadvantage significantly increased the likelihood of a variety of unsafe sexual behaviors and experiences. Low socioeconomic status not only increased female odds of exchanging sex for money or goods, it also raised female chances of experiencing coerced sex, and male and female odds of having multiple sexual partners in the year before the survey; it lowered female chances of secondary abstinence (practicing abstinence for a sustained period after becoming sexually active) in the year before the survey, female and male age at sexual debut, condom use at last sex, and communication with most recent sexual partner about sensitive topics. Low socioeconomic status has more consistent negative effects on female than on male sexual behaviors; it also raises the risk of early pregnancy. Controlling for wealth and other factors, orphanhood confers added risk for unsafe sexual behaviors. Poorer young people, especially females, also have access to significantly fewer media sources for family planning information. Without sufficient attention to local economic and social conditions in the design and placement of HIV-prevention programs, the potential effectiveness of the global response to HIV/AIDS is impaired.
The link between HIV/AIDS and women's property rights: whether violation of women's rights increases household poverty and women's own vulnerability to infection; and whether securing these rights can mitigate the impoverishing effect of the epidemic	Strickland 2004	Review	Women may be better able to prevent HIV infection or mitigate its consequences if their property and inheritance rights are protected. As illustrated by examples in several countries, these rights are often denied in practice. Differences exist between de jure and de facto rights to ownership and inheritance, and these need to be bridged. Some best practices in efforts to ensure women's property and inheritance rights are examined.

Interventions

Focus of the study	Author and date	Study design	Key findings and recommendations
How labor-saving technologies and practices can assist in overcoming labor shortages and how to promote their adoption and use by poor rural women in Kenya	Bishop-Sambrook 2003*	Cross-sectional study conducted in four communities in Bondo and Busia districts	HIV/AIDS causes labor shortages. Various initiatives are currently being undertaken in Bondo and Busia to help communities overcome labor constraints. These include conservation farming, tractor-hire services, and post-harvest and processing technologies. Constraints on adoption include lack of knowledge, information, cash, and time, a weak bargaining position, isolation of those affected, attitudes, and tradition. These technologies require inputs, time, and knowledge in the short term before they become effective. Recommendations are made in three areas: (1) increase farmers' exposure to new ideas and access to information; (2) develop appropriate skills and attitudes for the sustained use of labor-saving technologies and practices; and (3) increase farmers' access to relevant technologies.
Prioritizing HIV/AIDS prevention and mitigation activities in the face of severe financial and administration constraints	Ainsworth and Teokul 2000	Opinion	Where implementation capacity is weak, expanding the number of activities, as called for by multisectoral responses, may not improve effectiveness for the following reasons: (1) this approach calls for more interventions among more constituencies at a national scale, involving actors with even more limited capacity to act, which often have limited ability to realize their existing mandate; (2) these strategies are defined by the actors and scope of program, not by concrete, achievable outcomes; (3) there is a danger that the core activity—sustained behavior change among those most likely to contract and spread HIV—will continue to be shortchanged; (4) with increasing

(continued)

Interventions—Continued

Focus of the study	Author and date	Study design	Key findings and recommendations
			NGO involvement, governments may be marginalized. Recommendations include interventions to ensure behavior change among those with the riskiest behavior, ensuring universal access to treatment of opportunistic infections, and integrating AIDS into poverty-alleviation strategies in countries with generalized epidemics.
Pros and cons of microfinance in the context of HIV/AIDS	Parker et al. 2000*	Qualitative survey of about 30 microfinance institutions (19 of which participated in an extended dialogue) from various parts of Africa	Microfinance has three main limitations: (1) its scale—it serves only about two million clients across Africa; (2) an inherent tension between scale (the number of clients served) and scope (the extent of services provided to the clients); and (3) its inability to serve the neediest. Innovations in microfinance since the advent of HIV/AIDS include mandatory loan insurance, mandatory death-benefit insurance, legal services for participants, and education trusts for minors.
Enhancing understanding of HIV/AIDS mainstreaming; sharing experiences and strategies for mainstreaming HIV/AIDS practice	Elsey et al. 2003	Resource pack developed by a working group involved in HIV/AIDS mainstreaming in various sectors	Common strategies adopted by ministries to implement mainstreaming of HIV/AIDS strategies include use of research and impact and predictive studies; use of HIV/AIDS focal points; training; building structures for enabling high-level support; and influencing a wide range of actors and strategies, such as design and review of sector-wide approaches (SWAPs). Experiences with internal and external mainstreaming and potential process and impact indicators for mainstreaming are presented.
Significance of agricultural biodiversity and indigenous knowledge in the agricultural-sector strategy for HIV/AIDS	Gari and Villarreal 2002*	Participatory research in Uganda, Tanzania, Ethiopia, and Mali to identify agricultural responses relevant at the grassroots level	Use of traditional neglected and underutilized crops, agricultural diversification, home gardens, wild food plants, medicinal plants, and community seed systems should be promoted.

The role of labor-saving technologies in improving the food security of farm households in an HIV/AIDS context	Du Guerny 2004*	Conceptual	Labor-saving technologies should be introduced by (1) type of farming system and (2) type of farm household. As gender division of labor is intimately linked to functioning of farming household and system, special attention needs to be paid to gender issues when introducing these technologies.
Empirical evidence concerning the effects of AIDS on the agricultural and rural sectors and implications for agricultural policy; ways for governments and donors to assess and modify existing agricultural programs, policies, and investment strategies to take account of likely impacts of HIV/AIDS	Jayne et al. 2003	Review of literature and conceptual analysis	Agricultural policy can respond to the disease and contribute to its mitigation by focusing on investing in agricultural research to raise productivity of crop and livestock systems; rehabilitating public extension systems depleted by AIDS to disseminate the use of appropriate farming techniques; and instituting well-functioning crop and input marketing systems that contribute to small-scale farmers' productivity and food security.
Practical lessons on mitigating the impacts of HIV/AIDS through agriculture and rural development	HSRC 2003*	Workshop presentations and discussions	Interventions should combine development, relief, and rehabilitation, and policy should encourage and be influenced by realities in the community. Multisectoral partnerships at the district level are important, as is the need to move beyond labor-saving to labor-management. The report includes a summary of presentations, including "Study of practices implemented to mitigate the impact of HIV/AIDS at farm household level in six African countries" by Mike Connolly and "Mitigation of the impact of HIV/AIDS on livelihoods through low-labor input agriculture and related activities" by Tony Barnett and Rachel Grellier.
Experiences of development workers in mitigating the impacts of HIV/AIDS	White 2002*	Individuals who were involved in selected interventions were invited to write up their experiences. A list of questions was circulated to	The case studies reveal how existing development work can be reviewed and adapted in the light of knowledge of the impacts of HIV/AIDS on beneficiary families and communities (mainstreaming) and also how specific activities

(continued)

Interventions—Continued

Focus of the study	Author and date	Study design	Key findings and recommendations
		those who agreed to participate to assist them in focusing their analysis and producing a structured case study. Nine case studies were collected from projects in Uganda, Tanzania, Zimbabwe, and Lesotho.	can be devised to meet the particular needs of particular groups within communities. Many of the projects evolved from long-term development work and from consultation with community members. As most organizations in the study work in high-prevalence areas, distinguishing between those affected and unaffected by AIDS was unhelpful for targeting purposes. There are three core areas of intervention in livelihood activities: agricultural support and training, vocational training, and the provision of credit and loan schemes. Agricultural interventions such as promotion of year-round agricultural production, multiple farming systems, and technologies requiring low labor and other inputs are helpful. Vocational training projects need to be innovative. Credit and loan schemes need to be carefully designed to be responsive to local contexts. Lack of consistent monitoring and evaluation systems is a major drawback.
Evaluation plan for Intervention with Microfinance for AIDS and Gender Equity (IMAGE) program	IMAGE 2002	An integrated, prospective, randomized, controlled, community-matched intervention trial being conducted in the Sekhukhuneland region of South Africa's rural Limpopo province since late 2001. The primary study will compare information from individuals from villages that have access to IMAGE over a three-year period	IMAGE emphasizes the importance of the environment in which risky sexual behaviors, gender-based violence, and HIV infections are occurring. It combines the introduction of a poverty-targeted microfinance program to rural communities with a participatory learning and action curriculum (Sisters for Life) for clients. It plans to enroll 10 to 20 percent of households in targeted communities and to influence social norms, social networks and relationships, and community-level responses to issues such as poverty, gender-based violence, and HIV. The study is

		with those from villages that do not. IMAGE will be available to the control villages after the evaluation.	built around the prospective follow-up of three cohort pairs; IMAGE clients, young people living in the households of IMAGE clients, and young people living in communities where IMAGE is operating. Appropriate comparison groups are recruited from nonparticipating villages. Differences in key indicators (including gender-based violence, sexual behavior, and HIV) between groups from intervention and comparison communities will be analyzed.
Effect of HIV/AIDS on microentrepreneurs and their households; value of microfinance programs in helping clients mitigate the economic effects of chronic illness and death; what microfinance institutions can do to lessen the impact of HIV/AIDS on clients and on their organizations	Barnes et al. 2001	Survey of 338 clients of Zambuko Trust, an NGO in Zimbabwe providing credit and business management training, and 241 matched nonclient microentrepreneurs in 1997 and 1999. The survey was complemented by focus groups of Zambuko clients and staff. Respondents' households were characterized as HIV-affected using proxy indicators, such as chronic illness or death of an adult member or taking in orphans or sick persons.	In HIV-affected households, monthly income was Z$535 less than that of nonaffected households; the proportion of household members who were not economically active was greater; and household members were less likely to seek medical treatment because of lack of funds. Profits from enterprises declined among both clients and nonclients affected by HIV between 1997 and 1999 compared with unaffected clients and nonclients. Compared with HIV-affected nonclients, the HIV-affected client households had more sources of income; a significantly greater proportion of boys aged 6 through 16 were attending school; and 16 percent more clients had an individual savings account with a formal institution. At the end of 2000, about 0.3 percent of the Zambuko's outstanding loans were written off because of borrowers' death and illness. Measures taken by Zambuko to reduce the impact of death on its financial portfolio include a mandatory insurance fee of 1 percent to cover the loan if the client dies, a mandatory savings requirement, a policy of lending only to economically active clients, and strict enforcement of group coguarantees of loan installments.

(continued)

Interventions—Continued

Focus of the study	Author and date	Study design	Key findings and recommendations
Identification and analysis of effective mitigation practices; strategies for implementing and replicating such practices	Connolly 2003*	Literature review and field visits	Examples studied include pit farming and participatory impact monitoring in Zambia; a community program promoting healthy living through food and nutrition security in Zimbabwe; and community-based food banks in Malawi. More coordination of responses is needed among the micro, meso, and district levels so that insights can be translated into community action. The most effective and promising approaches to mitigation focus on participatory and group problem-solving approaches. Competent facilitation is needed, as is a paradigm change from the traditional transfer of agricultural technology to innovation and development in the community. A local community action cycle can help build a sense of ownership and the capacity of a community to respond effectively.
Sharing promising multisectoral practices and innovations for combating HIV/AIDS	AED (Academy for Educational Development) 2003	Compendium: organizations submitted descriptions of their practices in an agreed format	Twenty-two promising practices cutting across sectors were submitted by 13 organizations working in Africa. Most of these practices are relatively new and have yet to yield measurable results.
Three aspects of mainstreaming HIV/AIDS: in the workplace; in strategy and planning; and with focused interventions in HIV/AIDS	Mullins 2002	Synthesis of experiences in mainstreaming, mostly at Oxfam	Mainstreaming HIV/AIDS involves incorporating the issues surrounding the pandemic into all strategic planning and into day-to-day operations inside an organization, its programs, and its relationships with others. Organizations should anticipate and plan for likely problems arising from deaths and unexpected illness to avoid or minimize the impacts of HIV/AIDS. They should review and modify their overall strategies, program planning, and implementation. The impact of HIV/AIDS must be

			addressed on a sectorwide basis. Partnerships between organizations and HIV/AIDS specialists are beneficial. Mainstreaming HIV/AIDS needs to be a long-term, systematic process with a high level of commitment from senior managers and staff.
Integrating HIV/AIDS priorities into poverty-reduction strategies, including poverty-reduction strategy papers (PRSPs)	UNDP 2002	Policy guidance note	Integrating HIV/AIDS into PRSPs helps to create the necessary policy and planning environment for a comprehensive, multisectoral, and adequately funded response. UNDP and its partners must focus on nine policy areas as a matter of priority. A checklist with specific guidance on how to integrate or mainstream HIV/AIDS into PRSPs is provided.
Training at the country and subregional levels, encompassing NGOs and donor agencies; scaled-up HIV/AIDS programs in PRSPs and HIPC documents	UNAIDS/World Bank 2001	Toolkit	HIV/AIDS can be integrated into PRSPs and HIPC initiatives in the following ways: • Identify HIV/AIDS as a cause of poverty and include a discussion of poverty and income inequalities and their contributions to conditions that make people vulnerable to HIV infection and less able to cope with the consequences of being infected. • Situate the main strategies in the national HIV/AIDS plan as a central part of the overall national poverty reduction program, supplying justifications and costs. • Establish medium-term goals and poverty-monitoring indicators derived from the national HIV/AIDS plan. • Propose short-run actions for successful implementation of the national HIV/AIDS plan, with specific and measurable targets that form agreements for debt relief.

Annex 2: HIV/AIDS and Nutrition Evidence Base

Nutrition, HIV transmission, and disease progression

Focus of the study	Author and date	Study design	Key findings and recommendations
The relation between nutritional status and heterosexual HIV transmission in sexually active, adult women	Moore et al. 1993	A nested case-control study of sexually active, adult women in Kigali, Rwanda. Forty-five women who seroconverted during the 24-month study period were compared to 74 women who remained seronegative throughout the study.	Seroconverters and nonseroconverters did not differ in preseroconversion serum levels of vitamin A, carotenoids, vitamin E, selenium, albumin, ferritin, or cholesterol. Weight loss, however, was a significant predictor of eventual HIV seroconversion. Subsequent seroconverters lost an average of 1.5 kg during the first six months of the study, compared with 1.0 kg for nonconverters. Nine of 27 (33 percent) of seroconverters, compared with one of 44 (2 percent) controls, lost at least 5 kg in the six-month period beginning one year before their sero-conversion (odds ratio, 21.5). The association between weight loss and seroconversion was independent of other potential risk factors, such as socioeconomic status, pregnancy, and genital ulcer disease. In addition to these findings for measured weight loss during follow-up, reported weight loss before enrollment was a risk factor for subsequent seroconversion.
Effects of hormonal contraception, pregnancy, and vitamin A deficiency on cervical shedding in HIV-positive women	Mostad et al. 2000	A cross-sectional study of 273 HIV-positive women	Cervical shedding of herpes simplex virus (HSV) DNA was detected in 43 women (17 percent). Cervical shedding of HSV was significantly associated with oral contraception (adjusted odds ratio [aOR], 4.5), use of depo-medroxyprogesterone acetate (aOR, 3.2), and pregnancy (aOR, 7.9). In the subgroup of women who were not pregnant and not using hormonal contraception (n = 178), serum vitamin A was highly predictive of cervical HSV shedding: concentrations indicating severe deficiency, moderate deficiency, low-normal, and high-normal status were associated with 29 percent, 18

			percent, 8 percent, and 2 percent prevalence of cervical HSV shedding respectively.
Possible association of serum vitamin A levels with altered susceptibility to primary infection with HIV-1 in men engaging in high-risk sexual behavior with genital ulcers	MacDonald et al. 2001	HIV-1 seronegative men who presented for treatment at an STD clinic in Nairobi, Kenya, were prospectively followed. Vitamin A levels at study entry were compared between 38 men who seroconverted and 94 controls who remained seronegative.	Vitamin A deficiency (retinol <20 μg/dL) was present in 50 percent of HIV-1 seroconverters, compared with 76 percent of persistent seronegatives. Seroconversion was independently associated with a retinol level greater than 20 μg/dL (hazard ratio [HR], 2.43, 95 percent CI, 1.25 to 4.70, $P = 0.009$), and a genital ulcer etiology caused by *Haemophilus ducreyi* (HR 3.49, 95 percent CI, 1.03 to 11.67, $P = 0.04$). Circumcision was independently associated with protection (HR 0.46, 95 percent CI, 0.23 to 0.93, $P = 0.03$).
Timing and correlates of HIV-1 transmission through breast-feeding	Fawzi et al. 2002b	1,078 HIV-infected pregnant women from Dar es Salaam, Tanzania, enrolled in a trial to examine the effect of vitamin A and other vitamin supplements on mother-to-child transmission (MTCT) of HIV-1 and other health outcomes. Cumulative incidence was measured among children of women not randomized to vitamin A, given the higher risk of infection observed among those in the vitamin A arm. For analyses of correlates, data from all children not infected by age 6 weeks were used.	Mean duration of breastfeeding was 20.3 months. Thirty-seven infections were observed during 4,372 child-months of follow-up evaluation, or 10.2 cases per 100 child-years. Infection risk by age 4 months was 3.8 percent and increased to 17.9 percent by 24 months. In a multivariate proportional hazards model, high maternal viral load, low CD4+ cell count, and high maternal erythrocyte sedimentation rate were significant predictors of transmission of HIV-1 through breastfeeding. Mothers who had breast lesions during pregnancy were 2.00 times more likely to transmit the virus during breastfeeding than mothers without these lesions.
The relationship between maternal plasma RNA levels and mother-to-child transmission of HIV-1 in African breastfed children	Leroy et al. 2001	Nested case-control study within a randomized trial assessing the efficacy of a short maternal zidovudine (ZDV) regimen to reduce MTCT	At inclusion, mean log10 viral load was 4.6 among 55 transmitting mothers and 3.7 among 117 nontransmitters. Among transmitters, the mean difference in log10 viral load between day 8 postpartum and inclusion was –0.13 in the ZDV group ($n = 23$) versus 0.27 in the placebo

(continued)

Nutrition, HIV transmission, and disease progression—Continued

Focus of the study	Author and date	Study design	Key findings and recommendations
			group (n = 32); among nontransmitters, it was –0.35 for the ZDV group (n = 47) versus 0.27 in the placebo group. In multivariate logistic regression analysis, odds ratios for MTCT were 8.7 for 1 log(10) increase of maternal RNA at inclusion and 4.2 for 1 log(10) increase difference from inclusion to day 8 post-postpartum. High maternal viral load at inclusion strongly predicts MTCT of HIV in Africa. A short ZDV treatment regimen significantly reduces maternal viral load.
The effect of vitamin A on viral load	Coutsoudis et al. 1997	Pregnant women in Durban, South Africa, were enrolled in the study at between 28 and 32 weeks' gestation and received a daily capsule of vitamin A or placebo until delivery. The vitamin A capsule contained 5,000 IU of retinyl palmitate and 30 mg of beta-carotene. At delivery, each woman received 200,000 IU of retinyl palmitate to boost the vitamin A content of breast milk. None received any antiretroviral or steroid therapy.	Viral load did not increase in the treatment group after vitamin A treatment, although it increased significantly in the placebo group. The mean change in viral load was not statistically different between groups. Vitamin A supplementation is unlikely to increase HIV-1 replication in seropositive pregnant African women and attests to the advisability of continuing with vitamin A intervention trials to reduce MTCT of HIV-1 in developing countries. It also provides evidence that high-dose vitamin A supplementation given to lactating women (up to eight weeks postpartum) in populations at high risk for vitamin A deficiency is unlikely to increase the HIV viral load in those women who may be simultaneously HIV-infected.
The impact of single high-dose vitamin A supplementation, 60 mg retinol equivalent (200,000 IU), on HIV load and CD4 lymphocyte count	Semba et al. 1998	A randomized, double-blind, placebo-controlled clinical trial in Baltimore, Maryland. A group of 120 HIV-infected injection drug users were randomly allocated to	Vitamin A supplementation had no significant impact on HIV load or CD4 lymphocyte count at two and four weeks after treatment. This study suggests that high-dose vitamin A supplementation does not influence HIV load.

		receive vitamin A or placebo. Plasma vitamin A level, CD4 lymphocyte count, and HIV load were measured at baseline and two and four weeks after treatment.	
Effects of plasma, genital, and breast milk HIV-1 viral load and breast infections on perinatal HIV-1 transmission	John et al. 2001	A nested case-control study conducted within a randomized clinical trial of breastfeeding and formula feeding among HIV-1-seropositive mothers in Nairobi, Kenya	In analyses comparing 92 infected infants with 187 infants who were uninfected at two years, maternal viral RNA levels above 43,000 copies/mL (cohort median) were associated with a fourfold increase in risk of transmission. Maternal cervical HIV-1 DNA (odds ratio [OR], 2.4), vaginal HIV-1 DNA (OR, 2.3), and cervical or vaginal ulcers (OR, 2.7) were significantly associated with infant infection, independent of plasma virus load. Breastfeeding (OR, 1.7) and mastitis (relative risk [RR], 3.9) were associated with increased transmission overall, and mastitis (RR, 21.8) and breast abscess (RR, 51.6) were associated with late transmission (occurring more than 2 months postpartum). Use of methods that decrease infant exposure to HIV-1 in maternal genital secretions or breast milk may enhance currently recommended perinatal HIV-1 interventions.
The 24-month efficacy of a maternal short-course zidovudine regimen to prevent mother-to-child transmission of HIV-1 in a breast-feeding population in West Africa	Leroy et al. 2002	Data were pooled from two clinical trials conducted in Côte d'Ivoire and Burkina Faso between September 1995 and February 1998. Consenting HIV-1-seropositive women were randomly assigned to receive zidovudine or a placebo. Cumulative risks of infection were estimated using a competing-risk approach, with weaning as a competing event.	At 24 months, overall cumulative risk (CR) of MTCT was 0.225 in the zidovudine and 0.302 in the placebo group, a 26 percent reduction. Among children born to women with CD4 cell counts below 500 cells/μL at enrollment, CR of MTCT was similar in both groups: 0.396 in the zidovudine and 0.413 in the placebo group. Among children born to women with CD4 cell counts of 500 cells /μL or more, CRs of MTCT were 0.091 in the zidovudine and 0.220 in the placebo group, a 59 percent reduction. A maternal short-course zidovudine regimen reduces MTCT of HIV-1 at age 24 months, despite prolonged breastfeeding.

(continued)

Nutrition, HIV transmission, and disease progression—Continued

Focus of the study	Author and date	Study design	Key findings and recommendations
			However, efficacy was observed only among women with CD4 cell counts of 500 cells/μL or more.
Effects of vitamin A and multivitamins on birth outcomes in HIV-positive women in Tanzania	Fawzi et al. 1998	1,075 HIV-1-infected pregnant women between 12 and 27 weeks' gestation received (1) placebo or (2) vitamin A or (3) multivitamins excluding vitamin A, or (4) multivitamins including vitamin A in a randomized, double-blind, placebo-controlled trial with a 2 by 2 factorial design.	Multivitamin supplementation decreased the risk of low birth weight (<2,500 g) by 44 percent, severe preterm birth (<34 weeks' gestation) by 39 percent, and small size for gestational age at birth by 43 percent. Vitamin A supplementation had no significant effect on these variables. Multivitamins, but not vitamin A, resulted in a significant increase in CD4, CD8, and CD3 counts. Multivitamin supplementation is a low-cost way of substantially decreasing adverse pregnancy outcomes and increasing T-cell counts in HIV-1-infected women.
Whether hormonal contraceptive use, vitamin A deficiency, and other variables are risk factors for cervical and vaginal shedding of HIV-infected cells	Mostad et al. 1997	Between December 1994 and April 1996, women who attended a municipal STD clinic in Mombasa, Kenya, and had previously tested positive for HIV-1 were invited to take part in a cross-sectional study. Cervical and vaginal secretions from 318 women were evaluated for the presence of HIV-1.	Both cervical and vaginal shedding of HIV-1 infected cells were highly associated with CD4 lymphocyte depletion. After adjustment for CD4 count, cervical proviral shedding was significantly associated with use of depomedroxyprogesterone acetate (odds ratio [OR], 2.9), and with use of low-dose and high-dose oral contraceptive pills (OR, 3.8). Vitamin A deficiency was highly predictive of vaginal HIV-1 DNA shedding. After adjustment for CD4 count, severe vitamin A deficiency, moderate deficiency, and low-normal vitamin A status were associated with 12.9-, 8.0-, and 4.9-fold increased odds of vaginal shedding respectively.
Prevalence and correlates of HIV-1-infected cells in the genital tract	John et al. 1997	Cervical and vaginal secretions from HIV-1-seropositive pregnant women were evaluated.	Presence of HIV-1 DNA in the cervix was associated with cervical mucus and a significantly lower absolute CD4 cell count (354 vs. 469 cells/μL). An absolute CD4 cell count

			greater than 200 cells/μL was associated with 9.6-fold increased odds of cervical HIV-1 DNA detection compared with a count of 500 cells/μL or greater. Detection of vaginal HIV-1 DNA was associated with abnormal vaginal discharge, lower absolute CD4 cell count, and severe vitamin A deficiency.
Pathophysiology and epidemiology of mastitis and implications of mastitis in mother-to-child transmission of HIV	Semba and Neville 1999	Review	In many developing countries, transmission of HIV from mother to infant occurs through breastfeeding. Mastitis, an inflammatory process in the breast, can be common among lactating women in Africa and is associated with both higher HIV load in breast milk and MTCT of HIV. Antioxidant micronutrient deficiencies may increase the risk of mastitis.
Synthesis of the results of studies conducted examining the relationship between mastitis, HIV viral load in breast milk, and mother-to-child transmission of HIV	Semba 2000	Women in Blantyre, Malawi, were followed through second trimester and until children reached 12 months of age.	Among 334 HIV-infected women who were breastfeeding, the prevalence of mastitis, as indicated by elevated sodium levels in breast milk, was 16.4 percent at 6 weeks and 2.8 percent at 6 months postpartum. Mothers with mastitis had higher plasma viral load than mothers without mastitis, suggesting that more advanced disease may increase the risk of mastitis. Mastitis was associated with significantly higher MTCT rates at both 6 weeks and 12 months of age.
Prevalence and determinants of HIV-1-infected cells in breast milk	Nduati et al. 1995	Polymerase chain reaction (PCR) was used to analyze 212 breast-milk samples from 107 HIV-1-seropositive women.	Of the samples, 58 percent contained detectable HIV-1 DNA. Breast-milk samples with detectable HIV-1 DNA were more likely to be from women with absolute CD4 cell counts of less than 400 (odds ratio, 3.1). Severe vitamin A deficiency (<20 μg/dL) was associated with a 20-fold increased risk of having HIV-1 DNA in breast milk among women with CD4 counts below 400 cells/mm^3. Women with CD4 cell depletion, especially those with vitamin A deficiency, may be at increased risk of transmitting HIV-1 to their infants through breast milk.

(continued)

Nutrition, HIV transmission, and disease progression—Continued

Focus of the study	Author and date	Study design	Key findings and recommendations
The association between maternal HIV infection and perinatal outcome	Brocklehurst and French 1998	Systematic review of the literature and meta-analysis	The summary odds ratios of the risk of predefined adverse perinatal outcomes related to maternal HIV infection were as follows: spontaneous abortion, 4.05; stillbirth, 3.91; fetal abnormality, 1.08; perinatal mortality, 1.79; neonatal mortality, 1.10; infant mortality, 3.69; intrauterine growth retardation, 1.7; low birth weight, 2.09; and preterm delivery, 1.83. Sensitivity analyses showed that the association between infant mortality and maternal HIV infection was stronger in studies conducted in developing countries when compared with developed countries (odds ratios [OR], 3.72 and 8.6, respectively); studies of higher methodological quality compared with those of poorer quality (OR, 14.57 and 3.37 respectively); and studies that used restriction or matching to control for potential confounding factors compared with those that had not (OR, 11.60 and 3.35 respectively).
Predictors of vertical transmission of HIV-1	Fawzi et al. 2001	HIV-1-infected pregnant women were enrolled in a trial in Dar es Salaam, Tanzania, to examine the role of vitamin supplements. Intrauterine HIV-1 infection (HIV-positive at birth), intrapartum, and early breastfeeding transmission (HIV-positive at six weeks among those uninfected at birth) were determined using PCR.	Of 734 infants who had a specimen taken at birth, 62 were HIV-positive (8.4 percent). Of 367 infants who were uninfected at birth and were retested at 6 weeks, 59 infants were positive (16.1 percent). In multivariate analyses, maternal CD4 cell count, viral load, and clinical stage were significant predictors of both definitions of transmission. Viral load of 50,000 copies/mL or more at delivery was associated with a 4.21-fold increase in risk of transmission intrapartum and through early breastfeeding. Babies who were HIV-negative at birth and born before 34 weeks of gestation were 2.19 times more likely to become infected during intrapartum and early breastfeeding

			periods, compared with those born after 37 weeks. Gonorrhea at baseline was related to intrauterine but not intrapartum or early breastfeeding transmission. Signs of lower-genital infections at or after enrollment were also associated with transmission.
Sociodemographic, nutritional, immunologic, parasitic, and infant-risk factors for birth weight, low birth weight (LBW), and small-for-gestational-age (SGA) status in HIV-positive women in a clinical trial of vitamin supplementation and pregnancy outcomes	Dreyfuss et al. 2001	A cohort of 822 women in Dar es Salaam, Tanzania, were enrolled at prenatal care clinics during their second trimester, at which time blood, stool, urine, and genital specimens were collected, and anthropometric measurements and sociodemographic data were recorded. Birth weight was measured at hospital delivery.	In multivariate analyses, maternal weight at enrollment and a low CD8 cell count were inversely associated with LBW. Advanced HIV disease, previous history of pre-term birth, *Plasmodium falciparum* malaria, and any helminthic infection were associated with higher risk of LBW. The intestinal parasites *Entamoeba histolytica* and *Strongyloides stercoralis* were predictors of LBW despite their low prevalence in the cohort. In a multivariate-adjusted linear regression model, body mass index, mid-upper-arm circumference, a CD4 cell count of less than 200×10^6 cells/L (200 cells/mm^3), primiparity, maternal literacy, and infant HIV infection at birth were significantly associated with birth weight, in addition to risk factors included in the LBW model. Determinants of SGA included maternal weight, low serum vitamin E concentration, candidiasis, malaria, and infant HIV infection at birth.
Whether vitamin A prevents anemia, low birth weight (LBW), growth failure, HIV transmission, and mortality	Kumwenda et al. 2002	A controlled clinical study in Malawi that involved 697 HIV-infected pregnant women. Women received daily doses of iron and folate, either alone or combined with vitamin A (3 mg retinol equivalent), from between 18 and 28 weeks' gestation until delivery.	In the vitamin A and control groups, respectively, the mean (±SE) birth weights were 2895 ± 31 g and 2805 ± 32 g ($P = 0.05$),the proportions of LBW infants were 14.0 percent and 21.1 percent ($P = 0.03$), the proportions of anemic infants at six weeks postpartum were 23.4 percent and 40.6 percent ($P < 0.001$), and the respective cumulative proportions of infants who were HIV-infected at 6 weeks and 24 months of age were 26.6 percent and 27.8 percent ($P = 0.76$) and 27.7 percent and 32.8 percent

(continued)

Nutrition, HIV transmission, and disease progression—Continued

Focus of the study	Author and date	Study design	Key findings and recommendations
			(P = 0.21). Vitamin A improved birth weight and neonatal growth and reduced anemia but did not affect the rate of perinatal HIV transmission.
The effect of vitamin A supplementation to mothers on birth outcomes and mother-to-child transmission of HIV-1	Coutsoudis et al. 1999	A group of 728 pregnant, HIV-infected women received either vitamin A (368) or placebo (360) in a randomized, double-blind trial. HIV infection results were available for 632 children who were included in the Kaplan-Meier transmission analysis.	There was no difference in the risk of HIV infection by three months of age between the vitamin A (20.3 percent) and placebo groups (22.3 percent), nor were there differences in fetal or infant mortality rates between the two groups. Women receiving vitamin A supplement were, however, less likely to have a preterm delivery (preterm births were 11.4 percent in the vitamin A and 17.4 percent in the placebo group; P = 0.03) and among the 80 preterm deliveries, children of mothers in the vitamin A group were less likely to be HIV-infected (17.9 percent) than those in the placebo group (33.8 percent).
The efficacy of vitamin supplements in reducing HIV transmission through breastfeeding after six weeks of age and in child mortality in the first two years of life	Fawzi et al. 2002a	A total of 1,078 HIV-infected pregnant women in Tanzania were randomly assigned to receive either vitamin A or multivitamins excluding A from approximately 20 weeks' gestation throughout lactation.	Multivitamins excluding A had no effect on the total risk of HIV-1 transmission. Vitamin A increased the risk of transmission (RR, 1.38). Multivitamins were associated with statistically insignificant reductions in transmission through breastfeeding and in mortality by 24 months among those alive and not infected at six weeks. Multivitamins significantly reduced breastfeeding transmission in infants of mothers with low baseline lymphocyte counts (RR, 0.37) compared with infants of mothers with higher counts (RR, 0.99). Multivitamins also protected against transmission among mothers with a high erythrocyte sedimentation rate, low hemoglobin, and low-birth-weight babies. Multivitamins reduced death and prolonged

			HIV-free survival significantly among children born to women with low maternal immunological or nutritional status. Vitamin A alone increased breastfeeding transmission but had no effect on mortality by 24 months.
The effect of prenatal multimicronutrient supplementation on gestational length and birth size	Friis et al. 2004	A randomized, placebo-controlled, double-blind effectiveness trial among antenatal care attendees in Harare, Zimbabwe. Pregnant women (at 22 to 35 weeks' gestation) were randomly allocated to receive a multimicronutrient or placebo supplement daily until delivery. Supplementation with iron and folic acid was part of antenatal care.	Of 1,669 women, birth data were available from 1,106 (66 percent), of whom 360 (33 percent) had HIV infection. The mean gestational length was 39.1 weeks, and 16.6 percent of the women had a gestational length of more than 37 weeks. The mean birth weight was 3,030 g, and 10.5 percent of the infants had a birth weight of less than 2,500 g. Multimicronutrient supplementation was associated with tendencies for increased gestational length (0.3 weeks), birth weight (49 g), and head circumference (0.2 cm) but was not associated with low birth weight (less than 2,500 g) (relative risk, 0.84). The effect of multimicronutrient supplementation on birth weight was not significantly different between HIV-uninfected (26 g) and HIV-infected (101 g) subjects. Antenatal multimicronutrient supplementation may be one strategy for increasing birth size.
Vitamin A status in pregnant women as a risk factor for mother-to-child transmission of HIV	Semba et al. 1994	Serum vitamin A, height, weight, CD4 T-cell counts, and duration of breastfeeding were measured in 338 HIV-positive mothers in Malawi whose infants' HIV serostatus was known.	MTCT of HIV was 21.9 percent among mothers whose infants survived to 12 months of age. Mean vitamin A concentration in 74 mothers who transmitted HIV to their infants was lower than that in 264 mothers who did not transmit HIV to their infants (0.86 vs. 1.07 μmol/L). HIV-positive mothers were divided into four groups: those with vitamin A concentrations of less than 0.70 μmol/L, between 0.70 and 1.05, between 1.05 and 1.40, and 1.40 or more. The MTCT rates for each group were 32.4 percent, 26.2 percent, 16.0 percent, and 7.2 percent respectively. Low CD4 cell counts (and percentage) and

(continued)

Nutrition, HIV transmission, and disease progression—Continued

Focus of the study	Author and date	Study design	Key findings and recommendations
			low CD4/CD8 ratio were also associated with higher rates of MTCT. Maternal age, body-mass index, and breast-feeding practices were not significantly associated with rates of MTCT.
Role of vitamin A deficiency in mother-to-child HIV transmission	Greenberg et al. 1997	Third-trimester serum vitamin A levels were evaluated in 133 HIV-infected women in two U.S. cities who delivered live babies between 1986 and 1994 and whose infants' HIV status was known.	In a multivariate logistic regression model, severe vitamin A deficiency, Cesarean-section delivery, and prematurity were associated with MTCT after adjusting for CD4+ percentage and duration of membrane rupture.
The impact of malnutrition on survival in AIDS	Kotler et al. 1989	Body cell mass was evaluated by examining the magnitude of body-cell-mass depletion as a function of time from death. Body cell mass was estimated as total body potassium content and determined by whole-body counting.	There was progressive depletion of body-cell mass as patients neared death. The extrapolated and observed values for body cell mass at death were 54 percent of normal. Body weight had a similar relationship to death, with a projected body weight at death of 66 percent of ideal. Death from wasting in AIDS is related to the magnitude of tissue depletion and is independent of the underlying cause of wasting. The degree of wasting seen in this study is similar to historical reports of semi-starvation, with or without associated infections. This observation suggests that successful attempts to maintain body mass could prolong survival in patients with AIDS.
Association of mild weight loss with increased risk of death from HIV or opportunistic infections	Wheeler et al. 1998	A group of 2,382 participants from four interventional studies from a community-based clinical trials network were evaluated.	Weight loss of 5 to 10 percent is associated with an increased risk of opportunistic infections and complications. Weight loss of 5 percent over a period of four months is associated with an increased risk of death and opportunistic infections and complications.

Incidence and possible association of malnutrition and wasting with immunologic impairment; prognostic value of nutritional status	Suttmann et al. 1995	Nutritional, clinical, and immunologic parameters were measured in 100 outpatients in different stages of HIV infection. In addition, 39 patients with AIDS were prospectively followed for a mean period of 343 (range, 53–650) days.	Sixty-three percent of the patients showed evidence of malnutrition; 21 percent suffered from wasting. Reduced body cell mass and decreased serum albumin levels were observed in 32 and 14 percent of patients respectively, predominantly among those in more advanced stages of the disease. Fourteen of 39 AIDS patients died after a mean survival of 212 days. Survivors showed significantly larger initial body cell mass values and higher initial serum albumin levels than nonsurvivors, whereas CD4+ lymphocyte counts, disease complications, and medication were similar in both groups. Kaplan-Meier analyses revealed a significantly prolonged survival in patients with a body cell mass greater than 30 percent of body weight or serum albumin levels exceeding 30 g/L. Factor analyses indicated that the parameters of nutritional status were independent from each other and from CD4+ lymphocyte counts. Malnutrition occurs frequently during HIV infection and increases with disease progress. It strongly predicts patient survival independent of CD4+ lymphocyte counts.
Determining the prevalence of malnutrition in new tuberculosis (TB) patients and the association between malnutrition and early mortality (defined as death within the first four weeks of treatment)	Zachariah et al. 2002	New patients registered with TB in a rural district of Malawi were enrolled to determine (1) the prevalence of malnutrition on admission and (2) the association between malnutrition and early mortality.	Among 1,181 patients with TB (576 men and 605 women), the overall rate of infection with HIV was 80 percent. Of these, 673 (57 percent) were malnourished on admission (body-mass index of less than 18.5 kg/m^2). Ninety-five patients (8 percent) died during the first four weeks. Significant risk factors for early mortality included increasing degrees of malnutrition, age of more than 35 years, and HIV seropositivity. Of the 414 patients with moderate to severe malnutrition, 10.9 percent died in the first four weeks, compared with 6.5 percent of the 767 patients with normal to mild malnutrition (odds ratio, 1.8). In patients with TB, BMI below 17.0 kg/m^2 is associated with an increased risk of early death.

(continued)

Nutrition, HIV transmission, and disease progression—Continued

Focus of the study	Author and date	Study design	Key findings and recommendations
The effect of perinatally acquired HIV on somatic growth; the relationship of nutritional status and mortality in HIV-infected infants	Berhane et al. 1997	Pregnant women attending the antenatal clinic at Mulago hospital in Kampala, Uganda, were enrolled. All babies born alive to HIV-1 seropositive women, and to every fourth age-matched HIV-1 seronegative woman, were followed for 25 months.	The mean weight-for-age and length-for-age curves of HIV-positive children were significantly lower than those of HIV controls and seroeverters. Forty-five (54 percent) of the 84 HIV-positive infants died before their second birthday, as compared with 1.6 percent and 5.6 percent in HIV-negative infants and seroeverters. HIV-positive infants with an average weight-for-age z-score below –1.5 in the first year of life have a nearly fivefold higher risk of dying before 25 months of age than noninfected controls. Perinatally acquired HIV infection is associated with early and progressive growth failure. The severity of growth failure is associated with an increased risk of mortality.
The relationship between wasting syndrome and HIV seropositivity	Tang 2003	Review of data from the Tufts Nutrition for Healthy Living study	Analysis of Cox proportional hazards models showed that losses in weight, fat-free mass, body cell mass, and fat mass, both from baseline weight and from weight at previous follow-up, were all significant indicators of mortality in patients with HIV wasting syndrome. In the second analysis, the prevalence of 5 percent weight loss from the previous visit was shown to be 35 percent greater in the late HAART (highly active antiretroviral therapy) era, from 1998 to 2003, than in the early HAART era of 1995 to 1997. This corresponds with earlier observations that the diagnosis of HIV wasting increased during the 1990s. In the third analysis, the researchers found that body weight, fat-free mass, and body-mass index were better in patients receiving nutritional intervention than in patients receiving a placebo.

Association between different levels of dietary intake of micronutrients and progression of HIV-1 infection to AIDS	Tang et al. 1993	281 HIV-1-positive homosexual and bisexual men in the Multicenter AIDS Cohort Study completed a self-administered, semiquantitative food-frequency questionnaire at baseline. Levels of daily micronutrient intake at baseline were examined in relation to subsequent progression to AIDS during a median follow-up period of 6.8 years.	The highest levels of total intake (from food and supplements) of vitamins C and B1 and niacin were associated with a significantly decreased rate of progression to AIDS. The relation between total vitamin A intake and progression to AIDS appeared to be U-shaped; the lowest and highest quartiles of intake did most poorly, while the middle two quartiles were associated with significantly slower progression to AIDS (relative hazard [RH] = 0.55). Increased intake of zinc was monotonically and significantly associated with an increased risk of progression to AIDS (for highest vs. lowest quartiles, RH = 2.06). In a final multinutrient model, vitamin A, niacin, and zinc remained significantly associated with progression to AIDS, while vitamin C was only marginally significant.
The relation between dietary and supplemental micronutrient intake and subsequent mortality	Tang, Graham, and Saah 1996	Levels of daily micronutrient intake of participants in the Multicenter Acquired Immunodeficiency Syndrome Cohort Study were examined in relation to subsequent mortality over the eight-year follow-up period.	The highest quartile of intake for each B-group vitamin was independently associated with improved survival. In a final model, the third quartile of beta-carotene intake (RH = 0.60) was associated with improved survival, while increasing intakes of zinc were associated with poorer survival. Intakes of B6 supplements at more than twice the recommended dietary allowance were associated with improved survival (RH = 0.60), while intakes of B1 and B2 supplements at levels greater than five times the recommended dietary allowance were associated with improved survival. Any intake of zinc supplements was associated with poorer survival (RH = 1.49).
The associations between serum vitamin A and E levels and risk of progression to three key outcomes in HIV-1 infection: first AIDS diagnosis, CD4 cell decline to less than 200 cells/μL, and mortality	Tang et al. 1997a	Prospective study. Serum levels of vitamins A and E were measured at the enrollment visit of 311 HIV-seroprevalent homosexual and bisexual men participating in the Baltimore–Washington, D.C., site	Men in the highest quartile of serum vitamin E levels (≤23.5 μmol/L) showed a 34 percent decrease in risk of progression to AIDS compared with those in the lowest quartile (RH, 0.66). This effect was statistically significant when the highest quartile of serum vitamin E was compared to the remainder of the cohort (RH, 0.67).

(continued)

Nutrition, HIV transmission, and disease progression—Continued

Focus of the study	Author and date	Study design	Key findings and recommendations
		of the Multicenter AIDS Cohort Study. Cox proportional hazards models were used to estimate the relative hazard of progression to each outcome over the subsequent 9 years, adjusting for several independent covariates.	Associations between serum vitamin A levels and risk of progression to AIDS were less clear, but vitamin A levels were uniformly in the normal to high range. Similar trends were observed for each vitamin with regard to mortality, but neither vitamin was associated with CD4+ cell decline to less than 200 cells/µL. Men who reported current use of multivitamin or single vitamin E supplements had significantly higher serum tocopherol levels than those who were not taking supplements ($P = 0.0001$). Serum retinol levels were unrelated to intake of multivitamin or single vitamin A supplements.
The associations between serum concentrations of vitamin B6, vitamin B12, and folate and the risk of progression to first AIDS diagnosis and CD4+ cell decline to less than 200 cells/µL	Tang et al. 1997b	Prospective cohort study. The study population was drawn from a cohort of homosexual and bisexual men in the Baltimore–Washington, D.C., area. Eligible subjects were HIV-1-seropositive at study entry and had serum available in the serum repository from their 1984 baseline study visit. Serum micronutrient levels were assessed in 310 subjects. The follow-up period was approximately 9 years.	In Kaplan-Meier analyses, participants with low serum vitamin B12 concentrations (<120 pmol/L) had significantly shorter median AIDS-free time than those with adequate vitamin B12 concentrations (4 years and 8 years, respectively, $P = 0.004$). This effect persisted in Cox proportional hazards models after adjusting for HIV-1-related symptoms, CD4+ cell count, age, serum albumin, use of antiretroviral therapy before AIDS, and frequency of alcohol consumption (RH = 1.89). In additional analyses excluding subjects with more advanced disease at baseline, the increase in risk of progression to AIDS for those with low serum vitamin B12 concentrations remained significant (RH = 2.21), providing further evidence that low vitamin B12 concentrations preceded disease progression. In contrast, low serum concentrations of vitamin B6 and folate were not associated with either progression to AIDS or decline in CD4+ lymphocyte count.

The effects of daily supplements of vitamin A (preformed vitamin A and beta-carotene), multivitamins (vitamins B, C, and E), or both on progression of HIV disease, using survival models	Fawzi et al. 2004	The study enrolled 1,078 pregnant women infected with HIV in a double-blind, placebo-controlled trial in Dar es Salaam, Tanzania. The median follow-up with respect to survival was 71 months (interquartile range, 46 to 80).	Of 271 women who received multivitamins, 67 progressed to WHO stage 4 disease or died—the primary outcome—compared with 83 of 267 women who received placebo (24.7 percent vs. 31.1 percent; relative risk, 0.71). This regimen was also associated with reductions in the relative risk of death related to AIDS (0.73), progression to WHO stage 4 (0.50), and progression to stage 3 or higher (0.72). Multivitamins also resulted in significantly higher CD4+ and CD8+ cell counts and significantly lower viral loads. The effects of receiving vitamin A alone were smaller and for the most part not significantly different from those of receiving a placebo. Adding vitamin A to the multivitamin regimen reduced the benefit with regard to some of the end points examined. Multivitamin supplements delay the progression of HIV disease and provide an effective, low-cost means of delaying the initiation of antiretroviral therapy in HIV-infected women.
The effect of antioxidant vitamin supplementation on lipid peroxidation (a measure of oxidative stress) and viral load in humans	Allard et al. 1998	Forty-nine HIV-positive patients were randomized to receive supplements of both DL-alpha-tocopherol acetate (800 IU daily) and vitamin C (1,000 mg daily), or matched placebo, for three months.	The vitamin group (n = 26) had an increase in plasma concentrations of alpha-tocopherol ($P < 0.0005$) and vitamin C ($P < 0.005$) and a reduction in lipid peroxidation, as measured by breath pentane ($P < 0.025$), plasma lipid peroxides ($P < 0.01$), and malondialdehyde ($P < 0.0005$) when compared with controls (n = 23). There was also a trend toward a reduction in viral load (mean $\pm$ SD changes over three months, –0.45 $\pm$ 0.39 versus +0.50 $\pm$ 0.40 log10 copies/mL; $P = 0.1$; 95 percent confidence interval, –0.21 to –2.14). Nine infections were reported in the vitamin group and seven in the placebo group.

(continued)

Nutrition, HIV transmission, and disease progression—Continued

Focus of the study	Author and date	Study design	Key findings and recommendations
The effect of vitamin supplements in human immunodeficiency virus–infected, lactating mothers on child morbidity and CD4+ cell counts	Fawzi et al. 2003	A total of 1,078 HIV-1-infected women from Tanzania participated in a randomized, placebo-controlled trial using a factorial design to examine the effects of supplementation with vitamin A (preformed vitamin A and beta-carotene) and/or multivitamins. Supplements were given during pregnancy and lactation.	Children of women in the multivitamin groups had a significantly lower risk of diarrhea than did those in the no-multivitamin group. The mean CD4+ cell count was 151 cells/µL higher among children in the multivitamin groups than among those in the no-multivitamin group. HIV-positive children experienced a benefit apparently similar to that in HIV-negative children. Maternal receipt of vitamin A significantly reduced the risk that the child would have cough with a rapid respiratory rate, a proxy for pneumonia, but vitamin A had no effect on diarrhea or CD4+ cell count.
The relationship between selenium deficiency and mortality in HIV-1 disease	Baum and Shor-Posner 1998	Review	Selenium deficiency has been demonstrated to be a significant predictor of HIV-related mortality, independent of CD4 over time, CD4 below 200 cells/µL at baseline, and antiretroviral treatment. Although selenium deficiency in healthy humans is relatively rare, a number of studies have documented a decline in plasma selenium levels and decreased glutathione peroxidase activity in individuals with HIV/AIDS. These findings are of particular concern in light of selenium's influence on immune function, viral replication, and survival. As recent investigations indicate that supplementation with selenium may help to increase the enzymatic defense systems in HIV-infected patients, further studies to determine possible mechanisms and clinical trials to evaluate the effect of selenium supplementation on HIV disease progression are essential.

The role of nutritional status as a cofactor in HIV-related disease progression and survival	Baum 2000	Longitudinal follow-up of three distinct HIV-seropositive populations: 122 injection drug users (IDUs), 130 asymptomatic men who have sex with men (MSM), and 24 children	Nutritional deficiencies were widespread among all three groups, although the prevalence of nutritional alterations varied among the groups. Low levels of vitamin A, vitamin B12, zinc, and selenium were common and have been associated with disease progression and HIV-1 related mortality, independent of CD4 count of less than 200 cells/mm^3 at baseline and CD4 count over time. When all nutrient factors that are associated with survival are considered together, only selenium deficiency is a significant predictor of mortality. The profound effect of selenium on disease progression may reflect selenium's action in antioxidant defense systems as well as in gene regulation.
Vitamin A deficiency and wasting as possible risk factors for mortality from AIDS and infections	Semba et al. 1995	A nested case-control study within a large prospective cohort of HIV-infected injection drug users (IDUs). Fifty adult subjects who died from AIDS and infections were matched with 235 controls who survived. Plasma vitamin A, weight, and body-mass index were measured.	Mean length of follow-up was 2.4 ± 1.1 years. Vitamin A deficiency occurred in 50 percent and wasting in 38 percent of patients in the last visit before death. A CD4 cell count below 200/μL, wasting, and vitamin A deficiency were associated with mortality. There was a higher risk of death among HIV-infected subjects with vitamin A deficiency (odds ratio [OR], 4.6; 95 percent confidence interval [CI], 1.8 to 11.3) and wasting (OR, 8.8; 95 percent CI, 2.7 to 28.2). Vitamin A deficiency and wasting are common during HIV infection and are independent predictors of mortality in HIV-infected IDUs.
Whether clinical response to albendazole is improved by oral micronutrient supplementation	Kelly et al. 1999	HIV-seropositive patients with persistent diarrhea were randomized to albendazole plus vitamins A, C, and E, selenium, and zinc orally or albendazole plus placebo for two weeks.	Serum vitamin A and E concentrations before treatment were powerful predictors of early mortality, but supplementation did not reduce duration of diarrhea or mortality during the first month, even after taking into account initial vitamin A or E concentrations, CD4 cell count, or clinical markers of illness severity. Serum concentrations of vitamins A and E did not increase significantly in supplemented patients compared with those given placebo, and there were no changes in CD4 cell count or hematological parameters. No adverse events were detected except those attributable to underlying disease.

ARVs and nutrition

Focus of the study	Author and date	Study design	Key findings and recommendations
Whether highly active antiretroviral therapy (HAART) reduces the occurrence of HIV-associated weight loss and wasting	Wanke et al. 2000	Cohort study using longitudinal analysis	Of the cohort, 33.5 percent (156 individuals) met at least one definition of wasting. More than 50 percent of the cohort were receiving HAART when they met one of the definitions of wasting.
Total and regional body composition in 203 HIV-positive men and women receiving HAART	McDermott et al. 2001	A cross-sectional analysis of a cohort study of nutrition and HIV infection. Body composition was studied by dual-energy X-ray absorptiometry in 203 men and 62 women.	HAART is associated with redistribution of fat mass from the legs to the trunk, despite no significant changes in total fat mass or weight. In men, HAART is also associated with a reduction in bone mineral content, suggesting that HAART increases the risk of central obesity and osteoporosis.
Association of wasting with decreased survival in patients receiving HAART; which parameter (weight, fat-free mass [FFM], body cell mass [BCM], or fat mass [FM]) is most strongly associated with mortality	Tang et al. 2002	Study population consisted of 678 HIV-positive participants enrolled in the Tufts Nutrition for Healthy Living study.	Despite the apparent benefits of HAART use in extending HIV-related survival, weight loss remains an independent predictor of mortality. Measurement of FFM or BCM, estimated using bioelectrical impedance analysis, does not add prognostic value.
The prevalence and predictors of weight loss in the era of HAART	Batterham, Garsia, and Greenop 2002	A cross-sectional study of 122 HIV-positive subjects	Among subjects, 40 percent reported lipodystrophy, and 40 percent had documented weight loss. Using forward stepwise logistic regression analysis, only viral load (VL) was significantly associated with weight loss when intake, CD4 T-cell count, lipodystrophy, and age were entered into the model with VL (log copies/mL). Every one-log increase in HIV VL was associated with an odds of weight loss of 1.58 ($P = 0.0008$). Weight loss is still common in the HAART era. HIV VL was the most significant predictor of weight loss in this sample. Inadequate dietary intake and self-reported lipodystrophy were not related to weight loss in this population.

Treatment guidelines for HIV-associated wasting	Polsky et al. 2004	Practice guidelines	Management strategies for patients with HIV-associated wasting must be implemented concurrently. These strategies are controlling viral load, maximizing immune competence, correcting any immediate causes of wasting, addressing any psychosocial issues, improving nutritional intake, and treating anorexia. Special attention must be given to patients who display depletion of body cell mass; early and aggressive intervention is required.
The effect of protease inhibitors (PIs) on plasma lipid levels	Cheseaux et al. 2002	A systematic retrospective survey of all plasma lipid levels recorded for children who had received ritonavir or nelfinavir between 1995 and 2001 in Switzerland	Administration of PIs was associated with a significant increase in plasma cholesterol levels, which was more pronounced with ritonavir. Cholesterol levels exceeded 10.0 mmol/L in 3 of 49 (6 percent) PI-treated children and culminated at 13.8 mmol/L.
The effect of highly active anti-retroviral therapy (HAART) on growth in children with HIV-1 infection	Verweel et al. 2002	Analysis of selected growth parameters, clinical data, and laboratory results as part of a prospective, open, uncontrolled, multicenter study to evaluate the clinical, immunologic, and virologic response to HAART consisting of indinavir, zidovudine, and lamivudine in children with HIV-1 infection	HAART has a positive influence on the growth of HIV-1-infected children. This effect is sustained for at least 96 weeks. Height and weight are favorably influenced in children in whom HAART leads to a reduction of the viral load of at least 1.5 log or to less than 500 copies/mL and to an increase in the CD4+ T-cell z-score. In contrast to observations in adults on HAART, BMI did not increase in all children effectively treated with HAART. BMI increased more in children at an advanced stage of infection and with poor nutritional status at baseline. Data from pre-treated and naive patients were difficult to interpret because the baseline characteristics of these two groups differed.
A syndrome of peripheral lipodystrophy, hyperlipidemia, and insulin resistance in patients receiving potent HIV protease inhibitor therapy	Carr et al. 1998	Cross-sectional study of HIV-infected patients either receiving at least one protease inhibitor ($n = 116$) or protease inhibitor–naive ($n = 32$), and healthy men ($n = 47$)	HIV protease inhibitor–naive patients had body composition similar to that of healthy men. HIV protease inhibitor therapy was associated with substantially lower total body fat (13.2 vs. 18.7 kg in protease inhibitor–naive patients; $P = 0.005$), and significantly higher total cholesterol and

(continued)

ARVs and nutrition—Continued

Focus of the study	Author and date	Study design	Key findings and recommendations
			triglyceride levels. Lipodystrophy was observed clinically in 74 (64 percent) protease inhibitor recipients after a mean 13.9 months and 1 (3 percent) protease inhibitor–naive patient ($P = 0.0001$). Fat loss occurred in all regions except the abdomen after a median 10 months. Patients with lipodystrophy experienced a relative weight loss of 0.5 kg per month, had significantly higher triglyceride, cholesterol, insulin, and C-peptide levels, and were more insulin-resistant than protease inhibitor recipients without lipodystrophy.
Food and nutrition implications of ART and how to manage their effects in resource-limited settings	Castleman et al. 2003	Review	Interactions between antiretroviral therapy (ART) and food and nutrition can affect medication efficacy, nutritional status, and adherence to drug regimens. Drug–food interactions consist of the effects of food on medication efficacy, the effects of medication on nutrient utilization, the effects of medication side effects on food consumption, and unhealthy side effects caused by medication and certain foods. As ART interventions scale up in resource-limited settings, addressing food and nutrition implications becomes a critical component of care and support programs and services.
Summary of single-dose studies that characterize the pharmacokinetics of indinavir sulfate, a protease inhibitor, and the effect of food in healthy volunteers	Yeh et al. 1998	Randomized controlled clinical trial	The effect of food on the absorption of indinavir varied with the type of meal ingested. Absorption of indinavir most likely occurs in the upper portion of the small intestine. In a fasting stomach, indinavir can be emptied rapidly and absorbed efficiently. Meals high in fat may delay gastric emptying and have a buffering and

			neutralizing effect, which results in a rise in the gastric pH and possible precipitation of the indinavir. These characteristics are predictive of the pharmacokinetics of this potent antiretroviral agent at the steady state.
Role of zinc in HIV stage 4	Mocchegiani and Muzzioli 2000	Review	Zinc supplementation, along with HAART, resulted in reductions and, at times, disappearance of recidivistic opportunistic infections.
The benefit of oral zinc supplementation as an adjunct to zidovudine (AZT) therapy for treating opportunistic infections in AIDS	Mocchegiani et al. 1995	Randomized controlled trial	The frequency of opportunistic infectious episodes in the 24 months following entry into the study was reduced after zinc supplementation in stage 4 subgroup C1 subjects (11 infections vs. 25 in controls) and delayed in stage 3 zinc-treated subjects (1 infection over 24 months vs. 13 infections in controls). The effect of zinc is restricted to opportunistic infections due to *Pneumocystis carinii* and *Candida;* no variations have been observed in the frequencies of cytomegalovirus and toxoplasma infections. These data may support the use of zinc as an adjunct to AZT therapy in AIDS pathology.
The duration of initial and successive HAART regimens in the clinical setting among 405 previously ART-naive HIV-infected patients	Chen et al. 2003	Patients were selected from the University of Alabama at Birmingham HIV Outpatient Clinic from 1 January 1996 through 9 October 2001	One-half of HAART discontinuations were due to events associated with ART toxicity, such as vomiting and nausea. Failure to reduce viral load and/or poor adherence were the most common causes of HAART discontinuation after ART toxicities. As the duration of a HAART regimen increased, the likelihood of an individual to have received multiple treatment regimens also increased. Having an opportunistic infection or a history of injection drug use were the only factors significantly associated with shorter regimen duration.

(continued)

ARVs and nutrition—Continued

Focus of the study	Author and date	Study design	Key findings and recommendations
Improving delivery of ARV treatment in regions with high rates of HIV infection	Weiser et al. 2003	Cross-sectional study of determinants of ARV treatment (social, cultural, and structural) using both qualitative and quantitative research methodologies	Financial constraints constituted the most significant barrier to ARV adherence (44 percent). Other principal barriers included: stigma (15 percent); travel or migration (10 percent); and medication side effects (9 percent).
Adverse effects of HAART, specifically metabolic abnormalities, such as dyslipidemia, diabetes mellitus, insulin resistance, lipodystrophy, and lactic acidosis	Montessori et al. 2004	Review	Although antiretrovirals are becoming more effective, they are simultaneously becoming more complex. All antiretroviral drugs have short- and long-term adverse effects. These adverse effects demonstrate the need to find ways to prevent them and to ensure adherence to the drug regimen.
The prevalence of low vitamin B12 and red-blood-cell folate (RBFC) concentrations; how to differentiate between those with deficiency and those with harmlessly low vitamin B12 using homocysteine (sHcy)	Remacha et al. 2003	The study evaluated prevalence of low vitamin B12 and RBCF in 126 HIV-infected patients receiving HAART.	Prevalence of low vitamin B12 was significantly lower in patients receiving HAART than in previously studied patients who did not receive HAART. Prevalence of low vitamin B12 decreased after the introduction of HAART.

Micronutrient variations in HIV/AIDS patients before and after HAART	Rousseau et al. 2000	The study evaluated the nutritional status and micronutrients in 44 patients over three years. The first nutritional evaluation was conducted in 1995, before HAART; the second was conducted in 1998, when most patients received HAART.	Selenium and zinc deficiencies are dependent on immune status and sex in HIV/AIDS patients. Other micronutrients do not seem to be influenced by the immune status in these patients. HAART reduces selenium and zinc deficiencies and may help avoid weight loss independent of the CD4 cell count.
To assess the effect of triple ART on body composition and nutritional status, and on the prevalence of malnutrition in a sample of HIV-infected patients	Schwenk et al. 1999	Two longitudinal cross-sectional studies (1996 and 1997)	Prevalence of malnutrition decreased by 30 to 50 percent between 1996 and 1997. Triple ART may protect HIV-infected patients from developing malnutrition. Whole-body bioelectrical impedance analysis (BIA) suggests an increase in appendicular body cell mass associated with improved ART.
Clinical features, etiology, and pathogenesis of lipodystrophy in patients infected with HIV (LDHIV)	Chen et al. 2002	Clinical review	Because protease inhibitors (PIs) are the most effective means of promoting long-term survival in HIV-infected patients and provide superior suppression of HIV, the benefits from continued use most likely outweigh the side effects, such as LDHIV, in many patients.

References

ACC/SCN 2000. *Fourth report on the world nutrition situation.* Geneva: Standing Committee on Nutrition, United Nations.

AED (Academy for Educational Development). 2003. *Multisectoral responses to HIV/AIDS: A compendium of promising practices from Africa.* Washington, D.C.

Agarwal, H. K., R. S. Rao, S. Chandrashekhar, and J. B. Coulter. 1999. Knowledge and attitudes to HIV/AIDS of senior secondary pupils and trainee teachers in Udupi district, Karnataka, India. *Annals of Tropical Pediatrics* 19 (2): 143–149.

Ainsworth, M., and D. Filmer. 2002. *Poverty, AIDS, and children's schooling: A targeting dilemma.* World Bank Policy Research Working Paper 2885. Washington, D.C.: World Bank.

Ainsworth, M., and I. Semali. 1998. Who is mostly likely to die of AIDS? Socioeconomic correlates of adult death in Kagera region, Tanzania. In *Confronting AIDS: Evidence from the Developing World,* ed. M. Ainsworth, L. D. Fransen, and M. Over. Brussels: European Commission.

Ainsworth, M., and I. Semali. 2000. *The impact of adult deaths on children's health in northwestern Tanzania.* Policy Research Working Paper 2266. Washington, D.C.: World Bank.

Ainsworth, M., and W. Teokul. 2000. Breaking the silence: Setting realistic priorities for AIDS control in less-developed countries. *Lancet* 356: 55–60.

Allard, J. P., E. Aghdassi, J. Chau, C. Tam, C. M. Kovacs, I. E. Salit, and S. L. Walmsley. 1998. Effects of vitamin E and C supplementation on oxidative stress and viral load in HIV-infected subjects. *AIDS* 12 (13): 1653–1659.

Allen, L., and Gillespie, S. 2001. *What works? A review of the efficacy and effectiveness of nutrition interventions.* Geneva: United Nations ACC/SCN and Asian Development Bank.

Alleyne, E. P., A. Kapungwe, and R. Kamona. 2001. *The impact of HIV/AIDS on agriculture extension organization and field operations in Zambia.* Draft.

Ambati, B. K., J. Ambati, and A. M. Rao. 1997. Dynamics of knowledge and attitudes about AIDS among the educated in southern India. *AIDS Care* 9 (3): 319–330.

Anand K., C. S. Pandav, and L. M. Nath. 1999. Impact of HIV/AIDS on the national economy of India. *Health Policy* 47 (3): 195–205.

Auvert, B., A. Buvé, B. Ferry, M. Caraël, L. Morison, E. Lagarde, N. J. Robinson, M. Kahindo, J. Chege, N. Rutenberg, R. Musonda, M. Laourou, and E. Akam. 2001. Ecological and individual level analysis of risk factors for HIV infection in four urban populations in sub-Saharan Africa with different levels of HIV infection. *AIDS* 15 (Supplement 4): 15–30.

Barnes, C., E. Keogh, N. Nemarundwe, and L. Nyikahadzoi. 2001. *Microfinance and households coping with illness and death in Zimbabwe: An exploratory study.* Washington, D.C.: Management Systems International.

Barnett, T. 1994. *The effects of HIV/AIDS on farming systems and rural livelihoods in Uganda, Tanzania, and Zambia.* Rome: FAO.

———. 2004. Editorial: The cost of an HIV/AIDS epidemic. *Tropical Medicine and International Health* 9 (3): 315–317.

Barnett, T., and P. Blaikie. 1992. *AIDS in Africa: Its present and future impacts.* New York: Guilford Press.

Barnett, T., and D. Topouzis. 2003. *FAO and HIV/AIDS: Towards a food and livelihoods security based strategic response.* Rome: Sustainable Development Department, FAO.

Barnett, T., and A. Whiteside. 1999. HIV/AIDS and development: Case studies and conceptual framework. *European Journal of Development Research* 11 (2): 200–234.

———. 2000. The Jaipur paradigm: A conceptual framework for understanding social susceptibility and vulnerability to HIV. *South African Medical Journal* 90 (11): 1098–1101.

———. 2002. *AIDS in the 21st century: Disease and globalization.* New York: Palgrave Press.

Barnett, T., J. Tumushabe, G. B. Bantebya, R. Ssebuliba, J. Ngasongwa, D. Kapinga, M. Ndelike, M. Drinkwater, G. Mitti, and M. Haslwimmer. 1995. The social and economic impact of HIV/AIDS on farming systems and livelihoods in rural Africa: Some experience and lessons from Uganda, Tanzania, and Zambia. *Journal of International Development* 7 (1): 163–176.

Barrett, C. B., and Reardon, T. 2000. *Asset, activity, and income diversification among African agriculturalists: Some practical issues.* Project report to USAID BASIS CRSP, University of Wisconsin, Madison, Land Tenure Center.

Basu, A., D. B. Gupta, and G. Krishna. 1997. The household impact of adult mortality, morbidity, and mortality: Some implications of the potential epidemic of AIDS in India. In *The economics of HIV and AIDS: The case of south and southeast Asia,* ed. D. E. Bloom and P. Godwin. Delhi: Oxford University Press.

Batterham, M. J., R. Garsia, and P. Greenop. 2002. Prevalence and predictors of HIV-associated weight loss in the era of highly active antiretroviral therapy. *International Journal of STD & AIDS* 13: 744–747.

Baum, M. K. 2000. Role of micronutrients in HIV-infected intravenous drug users. *Journal of Acquired Immune Deficiency Syndromes* 25 (Supplement 1): S49–S52.

Baum, M. K., and G. Shor-Posner. 1998. Micronutrient status in relationship to mortality in HIV-1 disease. *Nutrition Reviews* 56 (1 Part 2): S135–S139.

Bechu, N. 1998. The impact of AIDS on the economy of families in Côte d'Ivoire: Changes in consumption among AIDS-affected households. In *Confronting AIDS: Evidence from the developing world,* ed. M. Ainsworth, L. Fransen, and M. Over. Brussels: European Commission.

Beegle, K. 2003. *Labor effects of adult mortality in Tanzanian households.* World Bank Policy Research Working Paper 3062. Washington, D.C.: World Bank.

Beisel, W. R. 1996. Nutrition in pediatric HIV infection: Setting the research agenda. Nutrition and Immune Function: Overview. *Journal of Nutrition* 126 (Supplement 10) 2611S–2615S.

Berhane, R., D. Bagenda, L. Marum, E. Aceng, C. Ndugwa, R. J. Bosch, and K. Olness. 1997. Growth failure as a prognostic indicator of mortality in pediatric HIV infection. *Pediatrics* 100 (1): E7–10.

Bharat, S., and P. Aggeleton. 1999. Facing the challenge: household responses to HIV/AIDS in Mumbai, India. *AIDS Care* 11 (1): 31–44.

Bharat, S., P. Aggeleton, and P. Tyrer. 2001. *India: HIV and AIDS-related discrimi-*

nation, stigmatisation and denial. UNAIDS Best Practice Collection: Key Material. Geneva: UNAIDS.

Bhattacharjee, J., R. S. Gupta, A. Kumar, and D. Jain. 2000. Pre- and extramarital heterosexual behavior of an urban community in Rajasthan, India. *Journal of Communicable Diseases* 32 (1): 33–39.

Binswanger, H. P. 2000. Scaling up HIV/AIDS programs to national coverage. *Science* 288 (5474): 2173–2176.

Bishop-Sambrook, C. 2003. *Labor constraints and the impact of HIV/AIDS on rural livelihoods in Bondo and Busia districts, western Kenya.* Rome: International Fund for Agricultural Development/FAO.

Bishop-Sambrook, C., and N. Tanzarn. 2003. *The susceptibility and vulnerability of small-scale fishing communities to HIV/AIDS in Uganda.* Rome: HIV/AIDS Programme, FAO.

Black, R. E. 1998. Therapeutic and preventive effects of zinc on serious childhood infectious diseases in developing countries. *American Journal of Clinical Nutrition* 68 (Supplement 2): 476S–479S.

Bloom, D., and S. Glied. 1993. Economic implications of AIDS in Asia. In *Economic implications of AIDS in Asia,* ed. D. Bloom and J. Lyons. Delhi: Oxford University Press.

Bloom, D., and A. Mahal. 1996: *Economic implications of AIDS in Asia.* New York: Columbia University Department of Economics.

———. 1997. AIDS, flu, and black death. In *The economics of HIV and AIDS: The case of south and southeast Asia,* ed. D. E. Bloom and P. Godwin. Delhi: Oxford University Press.

Bloom, S. S., M. Urassa, J. Ng'weshemi, and J. T. Boerma. 2002. Community effects on the risk of HIV infection in rural Tanzania. *Sexually Transmitted Infections* 78 (4): 261–266.

Boerma, J. T., S. Gregson, C. Nyamukapa, and M. Urassa. 2003. Understanding the uneven spread of HIV within Africa: Comparative study of biologic, behavioral, and contextual factors in rural populations in Tanzania and Zimbabwe. *Sexually Transmitted Infectious Diseases* 30 (10): 779–787.

Booysen, F. le R., and M. Bachmann. 2002. *HIV/AIDS, poverty and growth: Evidence from a household impact study conducted in the Free State Province, South Africa.* Paper presented at the Annual Conference of the Centre for the Study of African Economies, Oxford, March 18–19.

Bota, S., G. Malindi, and M. Nyekanyeka. 1998. Factoring AIDS into the agricultural sector in Malawi, Ministry of Agriculture and Irrigation. Cited in D. Topouzis, *Addressing the impact of HIV/AIDS on ministries of agriculture: Focus on eastern and southern Africa* (Rome: FAO/UNAIDS, 2003).

Brocklehurst, P., and R. French. 1998. The association between maternal HIV infection and perinatal outcome: A systematic review of the literature and meta-analysis. *British Journal of Obstetrics & Gynaecology* 105: 836–848.

Brown, L. R., P. Webb, and L. Haddad. 1994. The role of labor in household food security: Implications of AIDS in Africa. *Food Policy* 19 (6): 568–573.

Bryceson, D. 1999. African rural labor, income diversification and livelihood approaches: a long-term development perspective. *Review of African Political Economy* 26 (80): 171–189.

———. 2000. Rural Africa at the crossroads: Livelihoods practices and policies. Natural Perspectives 52, Overseas Development Institute (ODI). http://www.odi.org.uk/nrp/52.html.

Bryceson, D., J. Fonseca, and J. Kadzandira. 2004. Social pathways from the HIV/AIDS deadlock of disease, denial and desperation in rural Malawi. Lilongwe, Malawi: RENEWAL (Regional Network on HIV/AIDS, Rural Livelihoods, and Food Security)/CARE Malawi.

Burger, H., and B. Weiser. 2001. Biology of HIV-1 in women and men. *Clinical Obstetrics and Gynecology* 44 (2): 137–143.

Carney, D., ed. 1998. *Sustainable rural livelihoods: What contribution can we make?* London: Department for International Development.

Carr, A., K. Samaras, S. Burton, M. Law, J. Freund, D. J. Chisholm, and D. A. Cooper. 1998. A syndrome of peripheral lipodystrophy, hyperlipidemia and insulin resistance in patients receiving HIV protease inhibitors. *AIDS* 12 (7): F51–F58.

Case, A., C. Paxson, and J. Ableindinger. 2004. Orphans in Africa: Parental death, poverty, and school enrollment. *Demography* 41 (3): 483–508.

Castleman, T., E. Seumo-Fosso, and B. Cogill. 2003. *Food and nutrition implications of antiretroviral therapy in resource limited settings.* Technical Notes 7. Washington, D.C: FANTA.

Caulfield, L. E., M. de Onis, M. Blössner, and R. E. Black. 2004. Undernutrition as an underlying cause of child deaths associated with diarrhea, pneumonia, malaria, and measles. *American Journal of Clinical Nutrition* 80 (1): 193–198.

Chen, D., A. Misra, and A. Garg. 2002. Lipodystrophy in human immunodeficiency virus–infected patients. *Journal of Clinical Endocrinology & Metabolism* 87 (11): 4845–4856.

Chen, R. Y., A. O. Westfall, M. J. Mugavero, G. A. Cloud, J. L. Raper, A. G. Chatham, E. P. Acosta, K. H. Taylor, J. Carter, and M. S. Saag. 2003. Duration of highly active antiretroviral therapy regimens. *Clinical Infectious Diseases* 37 (5): 714–722.

Cheseaux, J. J., V. Jotterand, C. Aebi, H. Gnehm, C. Kind, D. Nadal, C. Rudin, C. A. Lazarevitch, P. Nicod, and V. Mooser. 2002. Hyperlipidemia in HIV-infected children treated with protease inhibitors: Relevance for cardiovascular diseases. *Journal of Acquired Immune Deficiency Syndromes* 30 (3): 288–293.

Collins, J., and B. Rau. 2000. *AIDS in the context of development.* Social Policy and Development No. Paper 4. Geneva: UNRISD and UNAIDS.

Connolly, M. 2003. *Study of practices implemented to mitigate the impact of HIV/AIDS at farm household level in six African countries.* Paper presented at the workshop on Mitigation of HIV/AIDS Impacts through Agricultural and Rural Development, Human Science Research Council, Pretoria, South Africa, May 27–29.

Coutsoudis, A., and N. Rollins. 2003. Breast feeding and HIV transmission: The jury is still out. *Journal of Pediatric Gastroenterology and Nutrition* 36: 434–442.

Coutsoudis, A., R. A. Bobat, H. M. Coovadia, L. Kuhn, W. Y. Tsai, and Z. A. Stein. 1995. The effects of vitamin A supplementation on the morbidity of children born to HIV-infected mothers. *American Journal of Public Health* 85: 1076–1081.

Coutsoudis, A., D. Moodley, K. Pillay, R. Harrigan, C. Stone, J. Moodley, and H. M. Coovadia. 1997. Effects of vitamin A supplementation on viral load in HIV-1-infected pregnant women. *Journal of Acquired Immune Deficiency Syndromes & Human Retrovirology* 15 (1): 86–87.

Coutsoudis, A., K. Pillay, E. Spooner, L. Kuhn, and H. M. Coovadia. 1999. Randomized trial testing the effect of vitamin A supplementation on pregnancy outcomes and early mother-to-child HIV-1 transmission in Durban, South Africa. South African Vitamin A Study Group. *AIDS* 13 (12): 1517–1524.

Decosas, J., and A. Adrien. 1997. Migration and HIV. *AIDS* 11 (Supplement A): S77–S84.

Deininger, K., M. Garcia, and K. Subbarao. 2003. AIDS-induced orphanhood as a systemic shock: Magnitude, impact and program interventions in Africa. *World Development* 31 (7): 1201–1220.

de Vincenzi, I. 1994. Longitudinal study of human immunodeficiency virus transmission by heterosexual partners. *New England Journal of Medicine* 331: 341–346.

De Waal, A., and A. Whiteside. 2003. New variant famine: AIDS and food crisis in southern Africa. *Lancet* 362 (9391): 1234–1237.

DFID (Department for International Development). 2003a. *Agriculture and poverty reduction: Unlocking the potential.* London.

———. 2003b. UK's Call for Action on HIV/AIDS. London.

Donovan, D., L. Bailey, E. Mpyisi, and M. Weber. 2003. *Prime-age adult morbidity and mortality in rural Rwanda: Effects on household income, agricultural production, and food security strategies.* Research report. http://www.aec.msu.edu/agecon/fs2/rwanda/index.htm.

Dreyfuss, M. L., G. I. Msamanga, D. Spiegelman, D. J. Hunter, E. J. Urassa, E. Hertzmark, and W. W. Fawzi. 2001. Determinants of low birth weight among HIV-infected pregnant women in Tanzania. *American Journal of Clinical Nutrition* 74 (6): 814–826.

Drimie, S. 2003. HIV/AIDS and land: Case studies from Kenya, Lesotho and South Africa. *Development Southern Africa* 20 (5): 647–658.

Drinkwater, M. 1993. *The effect of HIV/AIDS on agricultural production systems in Zambia: An analysis and field reports of case studies carried out in Mpongwe, Ndola rural district and Teta and Serenje district.* Rome: FAO.

Du Guerny, J. 2002. *Meeting the HIV/AIDS challenge to food security: The role of labor saving technologies in farm households.* Bangkok: UNDP Southeast Asia.

Ellis, F. 1998. Household strategies and rural livelihood diversification. *Journal of Development Studies* 3 (1): 1–38.

———. 2000. Rural livelihoods and diversity in developing countries. Oxford: Oxford University Press.

Elsey, H., P. Kutengule, S. Holden, D. Kasangaki, R. MacCarthy, A. Ofori-Asumnadu, and S. Smart. 2003. *HIV/AIDS mainstreaming: A definition, some experiences and strategies. A resource developed by HIV/AIDS focal points from governments and those that have been working on HIV/AIDS mainstreaming.* Durban, South Africa: Health Economics and HIV/AIDS Research Division.

Engh, I. E., L. Stloukal, and J. Du Guerny. 2000. *HIV/AIDS in Namibia: The impact on the livestock sector.* Rome: SD Dimensions, FAO.

FAO. 2003a. Food Security and HIV/AIDS: An Update. Committee on World Food Security, 29th Session, Rome, 12–16 May.

———. 2003b. *HIV/AIDS and Agriculture: Impacts and Responses. Case Studies from Namibia, Uganda and Zambia.* Rome.

Farmer, P. 1999. *Infections and inequalities: The modern plagues.* Berkeley, Calif.: University of California Press.

FASAZ (Farming Systems Association of Zambia)/FAO. 2003. *Interlinkages between HIV/AIDS, agricultural production and food security: Southern province, Zambia.* Rome: Integrated Support to Sustainable Development and Food Security Program (IP), FAO.

Fawzi, W. 2003. Micronutrients and human immunodeficiency virus type 1 disease progression among adults and children. *Clinical Infectious Diseases* 37 (Supplement 2): S112–S116.

Fawzi, W. W., T. C. Chalmers, M. G. Herrera, and F. Mosteller. 1993. Vitamin A supplementation and child mortality: A meta-analysis. *Journal of the American Medical Association* 269 (7): 898–903.

Fawzi, W., G. Msamanga, D. Spiegelman, E. N. J. Urassa, N. McGrath, D. Mwakagile, G. Antelman, R. Mbise, G. Herrera, S. Kapiga, W. Willet, and D. Hunter. 1998. Randomised trial of effects of vitamin supplements on pregnancy outcomes and T cell counts in HIV-1-infected women in Tanzania. *Lancet* 351 (9114): 1477–1482.

Fawzi, W. W., R. L. Mbise, E. Hertzmark, et al. 1999. A randomized trial of vitamin A in relation to mortality among human immunodeficiency virus-infected and uninfected children in Tanzania. *Pediatric Infectious Disease Journal* 18 (2): 127–133.

Fawzi, W. W., G. Msamanga, D. Hunter, E. Urassa, B. Renjifo, D. Mwakagile, E. Hertzmark, J. Coley, M. Garland, S. Kapiga, G. Antelman, M. Essex, and D. Spiegelman. 2000. Randomized trial of vitamin supplements in relation to vertical transmission of HIV-1 in Tanzania. *Journal of Acquired Immune Deficiency Syndromes* 23 (3): 246–254.

Fawzi, W., G. Msamanga, B. Renjifo, D. Spiegelman, E. Urassa, L. Hashemi, G. Antelman, M. Essex, and D. Hunter. 2001. Predictors of intrauterine and intrapartum transmission of HIV-1 among Tanzanian women. *AIDS* 15 (9): 1157–1165.

Fawzi, W., G. Msamanga, D. Hunter, B. Renjifo, G. Antelman, H. Bang, K. Manji, S. Kapiga, D. Mwakagile, M. Essex, and D. Spiegelman. 2002a. Randomized trial of vitamin supplements in relation to transmission of HIV-1 through breastfeeding and early child mortality. *AIDS* 16 (14): 1935–1944.

Fawzi, W., G. Msamanga, D. Spiegelman, B. Renjifo, H. Bang, S. Kapiga, J. Coley, E. Hertzmark, M. Essex , and D. Hunter. 2002b. Transmission of HIV-1 through breastfeeding among women in Dar es Salaam, Tanzania. *Journal of Acquired Immune Deficiency Syndromes* 31: 331–338.

Fawzi, W. W., G. I. Msamanga, R. Wei, D. Spiegelman, G. Antelman, E. Villamor, K. Manji, and D. Hunter. 2003. Effect of providing vitamin supplements to human immunodeficiency virus-infected, lactating mothers on the child's morbidity and CD4+ cell counts. *Clinical Infectious Diseases* 36 (8): 1053–1062.

Fawzi, W., G. Msamanga, D. Spiegelman, R. Wei, S. Kapiga, E. Villamor, D. Mwakagile, F. Mugusi, E. Hertzmark, M. Essex, and D. Hunter. 2004. A randomized trial of multivitamin supplements and HIV disease progression and mortality. *New England Journal of Medicine* 351 (1): 23–32.

Filteau, S. M., G. Lietz, G. Mulokozi, S. Bilotta, C. J. Henry, and A. M. Tomkins. 1999. Milk cytokines and subclinical breast inflammation in Tanzanian women: Effects of dietary red palm oil or sunflower oil supplementation. *Immunology* 97: 595–600.

Fleming, D. T., and J. N. Wasserheit. 1999. From epidemiological synergy to public health policy and practice: The contribution of other sexually transmitted diseases to sexual transmission of HIV infection. *Sexually Transmitted Infections* 75: 3–17.

Floyd, S., A. C. Crampin, J. R. Glynn, N. Madise, A. Nyondo, M. M. Khondowe, C. L. Njok, H. Kanyongoloka, B. Ngwire, B. Zaba, and P. E. M. Fime. 2003. *The impact of HIV on household structure in rural Malawi.* Paper presented at the scientific meeting on Empirical Evidence for the Demographic and Socio-economic Impact of AIDS, hosted by the Health Economics and HIV/AIDS Research Division (HEARD), Durban, 26–28 March.

Fox, M. P., S. Rosen, W. B. MacLeod, M. Wasunna, M. Bii, G. Foglia, and J. L. Simon. 2004. The impact of HIV/AIDS on labour productivity in Kenya. *Tropical Medicine & International Health* 9 (3): 318–324.

Friis, H., E. Gomo, N. Nyazema, P. Ndhlovu, H. Krarup, P. Kæstel, and K. F. Michaelsen. 2004. Effect of multimicronutrient supplementation on gestational length and birth size: A randomized, placebo-controlled, double-blind effectiveness trial in Zimbabwe. *American Journal of Clinical Nutrition* 80 (1): 178–184.

Galvin, S. R., and M. S. Cohen. 2004. The role of sexually transmitted diseases in HIV transmission. *Nature Reviews: Microbiology* 2 (1): 33–42.

Gari, J. A., and M. Villarreal. 2002. Agricultural sector responses to HIV/AIDS: Agrobiodiversity and indigenous knowledge. Rome: FAO.

Gertler, P., S. Martinez, D. Levine, and S. Bertozzi. 2003. Losing the presence and presents of parents: How parental death affects children. Draft.

Gilborn, L., R. Nyonyintono, R. Kabumbuli, and G. Jagwe-Wadda. 2001. *Making a difference for children affected by AIDS: Baseline findings from operations research in Uganda.* New York: Population Council.

Gillespie, S. R. 1989. Potential impact of AIDS on farming systems: A case study from Rwanda. *Land Use Policy* 6 (4): 301–312.

———. 2004. *Scaling up community driven development: A synthesis of experience.* Food Consumption and Nutrition Division Discussion Paper 180. Washington, D.C.: IFPRI.

Gillespie, S., L. Haddad, and R. Jackson. 2001. HIV/AIDS, food and nutrition security: Impacts and actions. In *Nutrition and HIV/AIDS,* Nutrition Policy Discussion Paper 20. Geneva: United Nations SCN.

Greenberg, B. L., R. D. Semba, P. E. Vink, J. J. Farley, M. Sivapalasingam, R. W. Steketee, D. M. Thea, and E. E. Schoenbaum. 1997. Vitamin A deficiency and maternal-infant transmissions of HIV in two metropolitan areas in the United States. *AIDS* 11 (3): 325–332.

Greig, F. E., and C. Koopman. 2003. Multilevel analysis of women's empowerment and HIV prevention: Quantitative survey results from a preliminary study in Botswana. *AIDS & Behavior* 7 (2): 195–208.

Government of Uganda. 2003. The Uganda Food and Nutrition Policy. Ministry of Agriculture, Animal Industry and Fisheries and Ministry of Health.

GTZ (Deutsche Gesellschaft für Technische Zusammenarbeit). 1999. *Factoring HIV/AIDS into the agricultural sector in Kenya.*

Guinness, L., D. Walker, P. Ndubani, J. Jama, and P. Kelly. 2003. Surviving the impact of HIV-related illness in the Zambian business sector. *AIDS Patient Care and STDs* 17 (7): 353–363.

Gupta, G. R., D. Whelan, and K. Allendorf. 2003. Integrating gender into HIV/AIDS programmes: A review paper. Geneva: World Health Organization.

Gupta, I. 1998. Planning for the socioeconomic impact of the epidemic: The costs of being ill. In *The looming epidemic: The impact of HIV/AIDS in India,* ed. P. Godwin. Delhi: Mosaic.

Haddad, L., and S. R. Gillespie. 2001. Effective food and nutrition policy responses to HIV/AIDS: What we know and what we need to know. *Journal of International Development* 13 (4): 487–511.

Hallman, K. 2004. *Socioeconomic disadvantage and unsafe sexual behaviors among young women and men in South Africa.* Policy Research Division Working Paper 190. New York: Population Council.

Hart, C. E., J. L. Lennox, M. Pratt-Palmore, T. C. Wright, R. F. Schinazi, T. Evans-Strickfaden, T. J. Bush, C. Schnell, L. J. Conley, K. A. Clancy, and T. V. Ellerbrock. 1999. Correlation of human immunodeficiency virus type 1 RNA levels in blood and the female genital tract. *Journal of Infectious Diseases* 179 (4): 871–882.

Harvey, P. 2004. HIV/AIDS and humanitarian action? Humanitarian Policy Group Report 16. London: Overseas Development Institute.

Haslwimmer, M. 1994. *Is HIV/AIDS a threat to livestock production? The example of Rakai, Uganda.* World Animal Review 3–4, ed. D. Chupin. Rome: FAO.

Hawkes, S., and K. G. Santhya. 2002. Diverse realities: Sexually transmitted infections and HIV in India. *Sexually Transmitted Infections* 78 (Supplement 1): i31–i39.

Hayes, R. J., K. F. Schulz, and F. A. Plummer. 1995. The cofactor effect of genital ulcers on the per-exposure risk of HIV transmission in sub-Saharan Africa. *Journal of Tropical Medicine and Hygiene* 98:1–8.

Hira, S., S. Gupta, and P. Godwin. 1998. HIV infection in the workforce and its perceived impact on the industry. In *The looming epidemic: The impact of HIV/AIDS in India,* ed. P. Godwin. New Delhi: Mosaic.

Hope, K. R. 2001. Population mobility and multi-partner sex in Botswana: Implications for the spread of HIV/AIDS. *African Journal of Reproductive Health* 5 (3): 73–83.

Hosegood, V., K. Herbst, and I. Timæus. 2003. *The impact of adult AIDS deaths on households and children's living arrangements in rural South Africa.* Paper presented at the scientific meeting on Empirical Evidence for the Demographic and Socio-economic Impact of AIDS, hosted by the Health Economics and HIV/AIDS Research Division (HEARD), Durban, 26–28 March.

HSRC (Human Science Research Council). 2003. *Mitigation of HIV/AIDS impacts through agricultural and rural development: Success stories and future actions.* Workshop report, May 27–29. Pretoria, South Africa.

IFPRI (International Food Policy Research Institute). 2004. *A way forward from the 2020 Africa Conference: Assuring food and nutrition security in Africa by 2020. Prioritizing actions, strengthening actors, and facilitating partnerships.* Kampala, Uganda.

IMAGE. 2002. *Social interventions for HIV/AIDS : Intervention with micro-finance for AIDS and gender equity.* Evaluation Monograph 1. Rural AIDS Development Action Research Programme (RADAR).

Janjaroen, W. 1998. The impact of AIDS on household composition and consumption in Thailand. In *Confronting AIDS: Evidence from the developing world,* ed. M. Ainsworth, L. Fransen, and M. Over. Brussels: European Commission.

Jayne, T. S., M. Villarreal, and P. Pingali. 2003. *Interactions between the agricultural sector and the HIV/AIDS pandemic.* Rome: FAO.

Jewkes, R., and N. Abrahams. 2002. The epidemiology of rape and sexual coercion in South Africa: An overview. *Social Science & Medicine* 55 (7): 1231–1244.

John, G. C., R. W. Nduati, D. Mbori-Ngacha, J. Overbaugh, M. Welch, B. A. Richardson, J. Ndinya-Achola, J. Bwayo, J. Krieger, F. Onyango, and J. K. Kreiss. 1997. Genital shedding of human immunodeficiency virus type 1 DNA during pregnancy: Association with immunosuppression, abnormal cervical or vaginal discharge, and severe vitamin A deficiency. *Journal of Infectious Diseases* 175 (1): 57–62.

John, G. C., R. W. Nduati, D. A. Mbori-Ngacha, B. A. Richardson, D. Panteleeff, A. Mwatha, J. Overbaugh, J. Bwayo, J. O. Ndinya-Achola, and J. K. Kreiss. 2001. Correlates of mother-to-child human immunodeficiency virus type 1 (HIV-1) transmission: Association with maternal plasma HIV-1 RNA load, genital HIV-1 DNA shedding, and breast infections. *Journal of Infectious Diseases* 183 (2): 206–212.

Jones, S. G., and F. Holloman. 2000. Continuous quality improvement project: Decreasing the potential for the development in the inpatient setting of drug resistance by improving nursing practice for HAART administration. *Journal of the Association of Nurses in AIDS Care* 11 (2): 76–86.

Kadiyala, S. 2004. *Scaling up HIV/AID interventions through expanded partnerships (STEPs) in Malawi.* Food Consumption and Nutrition Division Discussion Paper 179. Washington, D.C.: International Food Policy Research Institute.

Kadiyala, S., and T. Barnett. 2004. AIDS in India: Disaster in the making. *Economic and Political Weekly* 39 (19): 1888–1892.

Kadiyala, S., and Gillespie, S. 2004. Rethinking food aid to fight AIDS. *Food and Nutrition Bulletin* 25 (3): 271–282.

Kanjilal, B. 1995. *Implications of HIV/AIDS epidemic on trucking industry.* Jaipur: Indian Institute of Health Management Research.

Kelly, P., R. Musonda, E. Kafwembe, L. Kaetano, E. Keane, and M. Farthing. 1999. Micronutrient supplementation in the AIDS diarrhoea–wasting syndrome in Zambia: A randomized controlled trial. *AIDS* 13 (4): 495–500.

Kotler, D. P., A. R. Tierney, J. Wang, and R. N. Pierson Jr. 1989. Magnitude of body-cell-mass depletion and the timing of death from wasting in AIDS. *American Journal of Clinical Nutrition* 50 (3): 444–447.

Kovacs, A., L. S. Chan, Z. C. Chen, W. A. Meyer III, L. Muderspach, M. Young, K. Anastos, and A. M. Levine. 1999. HIV-1 RNA in plasma and genital tract secretions in women infected with HIV-1. *Journal of Acquired Immune Deficiency Syndromes* 22 (2): 124–131.

Kumwenda, N., P. G. Miotti, T. E. Taha, R. Broadhead, R. J. Biggar, J. B. Jackson, G. Melikian, and R. D. Semba. 2002. Antenatal vitamin A supplementation increases birth weight and decreases anemia among infants born to human immunodeficiency virus–infected women in Malawi. *Clinical Infectious Diseases* 35 (5): 618–624.

Kwaramba, P. 1997. *The socio-economic impact of AIDS on commercial agricultural production systems in Zimbabwe.* Harare: Zimbabwe Farmer's Union and Friedrich Ebert Stiftung.

Lagarde, E., v. d. L. Schim, C. Enel, B. Holmgren, R. Dray-Spira, G. Pison, J. P. Piau, V. Delaunay, S. M'Boup, I. Ndoye, M. Coeuret-Pellicer, H. Whittle, and P. Aaby. 2003. Mobility and the spread of human immunodeficiency virus into rural areas of West Africa. *International Journal of Epidemiology* 32 (5): 744–752.

Lal, S. S., R. S. Vasan, P. S. Sarma, and K. R. Thankappan. 2000. Knowledge and attitude of college students in Kerala towards HIV/AIDS, sexually transmitted diseases and sexuality. *National Medical Journal of India* 13(5): 231–236.

Landesman, S. H., L. A. Kalish, D. N. Burns, H. Minkoff, H. E. Fox, C. Zorrilla, P. Garcia, M. G. Fowler, L. Mofenson, and R. Tuomala. 1996. Obstetrical factors and the transmission of human immunodeficiency virus type 1 from mother to child: The Women and Infants Transmission Study. *New England Journal of Medicine* 334 (25): 1617–1623.

Leroy, V., C. Montcho, O. Manigart, P. P. Van de, F. Dabis, P. Msellati, N. Meda, B. You, A. Simonon, and C. Rouzioux. 2001. Maternal plasma viral load, zidovudine and mother-to-child transmission of HIV-1 in Africa: DITRAME ANRS 049a trial. *AIDS* 15 (4): 517–522.

Leroy, V., J. M. Karon, A. Alioum, E. R. Ekpini, N. Meda, A. E. Greenberg, P. Msellati, M. Hudgens, F. Dabis, and S. Z. Wiktor. 2002. Twenty-four month efficacy of a maternal short-course zidovudine regimen to prevent mother-to-child transmission of HIV-1 in West Africa. *AIDS* 16 (4): 631–641.

Lewis, O. 1976. *Five Families: Mexican Case Studies in the Culture of Poverty.* New York: Basic Books.

Lipsky, J. J. 1998. Abnormal fat accumulation in patients with HIV-1 infection. *Lancet* 351 (9106): 847–848.

Loevinsohn, M., and S. R. Gillespie. 2003a. *HIV/AIDS, Food security and rural livelihoods: Understanding and responding.* Food Consumption and Nutrition Division Discussion Paper 157. Washington, D.C.: International Food Policy Research Institute.

———. 2003b. *HIV/AIDS and food crises in southern Africa: An agenda for action research and for learning how to respond.* RENEWAL working paper. http://www.isnar.org/renewal.

Long, E. M., H. L. Martin, J. K. Kreiss, S. M. J. Rainwater, L. Lavreys, D. J. Jackson, J. Rakwar, K. Mandaliya, and J. Overbaugh. 2000. Gender differences in HIV-1 diversity at time of infection. *Nature Medicine* 6 (1): 71–75.

Lundberg, M., and M. Over. 2000. Sources of financial assistance for households suffering an adult death in Kagera, Tanzania. *South African Journal of Economics* 68 (5): 1–39.

MacDonald, K. S., I. Malonza, D. K. Chen, N. J. Nagelkerke, J. M. Nasio, J. Ndinya-Achola, J. J. Bwayo, D. S. Sitar, F. Y. Aoki, and F. A. Plummer. 2001. Vitamin A and risk of HIV-1 seroconversion among Kenyan men with genital ulcers. *AIDS* 15 (5): 635–639.

Marston, B., and K. M. De Cock. 2004. Multivitamins, nutrition, and antiretroviral therapy for HIV disease in Africa. *New England Journal of Medicine* 351 (1): 78–80.

Mason, J. B., A. T. Bailes, and K. E. Mason. 2003. *Drought, AIDS and child malnutrition in Southern Africa.* Paper prepared for UNICEF Regional Office for Eastern and Southern Africa. New Orleans: Tulane University.

Mastro, T. D., and I. de Vincenzi. 1996. Probabilities of sexual HIV-1 transmission. *AIDS* 10 (Supplement A): S75–S82.

Mather, D., D. Donovan, M. Weber, H. Marrule, and A. Alage. 2004a. *Prime age adult mortality and household livelihood in rural Mozambique: Preliminary results and implications for HIV/AIDS mitigation efforts.* Reprint of paper prepared for the Annual Conference of the Centre for the Study of African Economies, Oxford, March.

Mather, D., D. Donovan, T. Jayne, M. Weber, E. Mazhangara, L. Bailey, K. Yoo, T. Yamano, and E. Mghenyi. 2004b. *A cross-country analysis of household responses to adult mortality in rural sub-Saharan Africa: Implications for HIV/AIDS mitigation and rural development policies.* Paper prepared for the International AIDS Economics Network Pre-Conference, Bangkok, Thailand, 9–10 July.

McCullough, F. S., C. A. Northrop-Clewes, and D. I. Thurnham. 1999. The effect of vitamin A on epithelial integrity. *Proceedings of the Nutrition Society* 58 (2): 289–293.

McDermott, A. Y., A. Shevitz, T. Knox, R. Roubenoff, J. Kehayias, and S. Gorbach. 2001. Effect of highly active antiretroviral therapy on fat, lean, and bone mass in HIV-seropositive men and women. *American Journal of Clinical Nutrition* 74 (5): 679–686.

Menon, R., J. M. Wawer, K. J. Konde-Lule, N. K. Sewankembo, and L. Chuanjun. 1998. The economic impact of adult mortality on households in Rakai district, Uganda. In *Confronting AIDS: Evidence from the developing world,* ed. M. Ainsworth, L. Fransen, and M. Over. Brussels: European Commission.

Millennium Project. 2004. *Interim Report: Halving Hunger by 2015: A Framework for Action.* New York: Millennium Project, Columbia University.

Mocchegiani, E., and M. Muzzioli. 2000. Therapeutic application of zinc in human immunodeficiency virus against opportunistic infections. *Journal of Nutrition* 130 (Supplement 5): 1424S–1431S.

Mocchegiani, E., S. Veccia, F. Ancarani, G. Scalise, and N. Fabris. 1995. Benefit of oral zinc supplementation as an adjunct to zidovudine (AZT) therapy against opportunistic infections in AIDS. *International Journal of Immunopharmacology* 17 (9): 719–727.

Mocroft, A., M. J. Gill, W. Davidson, and A. N. Phillips. 2000. Are there gender differences in starting protease inhibitors, HAART, and disease progression despite equal access to care? *Journal of Acquired Immune Deficiency Syndromes* 24 (5): 475–482.

Montessori, V., N. Press, M. Harris, L. Akagi, and J. S. G. Montaner. 2004. Adverse effects of antiretroviral therapy for HIV infection. *Canadian Medical Association Journal* 170 (2): 229–238.

Moore, P. S., S. Allen, A. L. Sowell, P. P. Van de Perre, D. L. Huff, A. Serufilira, F. Nsengumuremyi, and S. B. Hulley. 1993. Role of nutritional status and weight loss in HIV seroconversion among Rwandan women. *Journal of Acquired Immune Deficiency Syndromes* 6 (6): 611–616.

Morris, C., D. R. Burdge, and E. J. Cheevers. 2000. Economic impact of HIV infection in a cohort of male sugar mill workers in South Africa. *Journal of South African Economics* 68 (5): 933–946.

Mostad, S. B., J. Overbaugh, D. M. DeVange, M. J. Welch, B. Chohan, K. Mandaliya, P. Nyange, H. L. Martin Jr., J. Ndinya-Achola, J. J. Bwayo, and J. K. Kreiss. 1997. Hormonal contraception, vitamin A deficiency, and other risk factors for shedding of HIV-1 infected cells from the cervix and vagina. *Lancet* 350 (9082): 922–927.

Mostad, S. B., J. K. Kreiss, A. J. Ryncarz, K. Mandaliya, N. B. Chohan, J. Ndinya-Achola, J. J. Bwayo, and L. Corey. 2000. Cervical shedding of herpes simplex virus in human immunodeficiency virus-infected women: Effects of hormonal contraception, pregnancy, and vitamin A deficiency. *Journal of Acquired Immune Deficiency Syndromes* 181 (1): 58–63.

Mullins, D. 2002. *What can it look like to mainstream HIV and AIDS?* Pretoria: Oxfam UK.

Mutangadura, G. 2000. Household welfare impacts of mortality of adult females in Zimbabwe: Implications for policy and program development. Paper presented at the AIDS and Economics Symposium, organized by IAEN Network, Durban, July 7–8.

Mutangadura, G., D. Mukurazita, and H. Jackson. 1999. *A review of household and community responses to HIV/AIDS epidemic in rural areas of sub-Saharan Africa.* UNAIDS Best Practice Collection. Geneva: UNAIDS.

Muwanga, F. T. 2002. *Impact of HIV/AIDS on agriculture and the private sector in Swaziland: The demographic, social and economic impact on subsistence agriculture, commercial agriculture, Ministry of Agriculture, and Co-operatives and Business.* Swaziland: Ministry of Agriculture and Co-operatives and Business.

Mwakalobo, A. 2003. *Implications of HIV/AIDS on rural livelihoods in Tanzania: The case of Rungwe district.* Unpublished ms.

NAADS (National Agricultural Advisory Services). 2003. *The impact of HIV/AIDS on the agricultural sector and rural livelihoods in Uganda.* Rome: Integrated Support to Sustainable Development and Food Security Programme (IP), FAO.

NACO (National AIDS Control Organization). 2004. An overview of the spread and prevalence of HIV/AIDS in India. New Delhi. http://www.nacoonline.org/facts.htm.

Nampanya-Serpell, N. 2000. *Social and economic risk factors for HIV/AIDS-affected families in Zambia.* Paper presented at the AIDS and Economics Symposium, Durban, July 7–8.

Nduati, R. W., G. C. John, B. A. Richardson, J. Overbaugh, M. Welch, J. Ndinya-Achola, S. Moses, K. Holmes, F. Onyango, and J. K. Kreiss. 1995. Human immunodeficiency virus type 1-infected cells in breast milk: Association with immunosuppression and vitamin A deficiency. *Journal of Infectious Diseases* 172 (6): 1461–1468.

Newman, S., P. Sarin, N. Kumaraswamy, et al. 2000. Marriage, monogamy and HIV: A profile of HIV-infected women in south India. *International Journal of STD and HIV/AIDS* 11 (4): 250–253.

Nicolosi, A., M. L. Correa Leite, M. Musicco, C. Arici, G. Gavazzeni, and A. Lazzarin. 1994. The efficiency of male-to-female and female-to-male sexual transmission of the human immunodeficiency virus: A study of 730 stable couples. *Epidemiology* 5: 570–575.

Nilses, C., G. Lindmark, S. Munjanja, and L. Nystrom. 2000. A community based study of HIV in women in rural Gutu District, Zimbabwe, 1992 to 1993. *Central African Journal of Medicine* 46 (2): 32–37.

Noback, R. R., and Y. I. Takahashi. 1978. Micromorphology of the placenta of rats reared on marginal vitamin A deficient diet. *Acta Anatomica* 102: 195–202.

Ntozi, J. P. M. 1997. Widowhood, remarriage and migration during the HIV/AIDS epidemic in Uganda. *Health Transition Review* 7 (Supplement): 125–144.

Nyambedha, E. O., et al. 2001. Policy implications of the inadequate support systems for orphans in Western Kenya. *Health Policy* 58: 83–96.

Oni, S. A., et al. 2002. The economic impact of HIV/AIDS on rural households in Limpopo Province. *South African Journal of Economics* 70 (7): 1173–1192.

Palella, F. J., M. Deloria-Knoll, J. S. Chmiel, A. C. Moorman, K. C. Wood, A. E. Greenberg, and S. D. Holmberg. 2003. Survival benefit of initiating antiretroviral therapy in HIV-infected persons in different CD4(+) cell strata. *Annals of Internal Medicine* 138 (8): 620–626.

Pandav, C. S., et al. 1997. Economic consequences of HIV/AIDS in India. *National Medical Journal of India* 10 (1): 27–30.

Parker, J., I. Singh, and K. Hattel. 2000. *The role of microfinance in the fight against HIV/AIDS.* UNAIDS background paper. Bethesda, Md.: Development Alternatives.

Pelletier, D. L., E. A. Frongillio Jr., D. G Schroeder, and J. P. Habicht. 1994. A methodology for estimating the contribution of malnutrition to child mortality in developing countries. *Journal of Nutrition* 124: 2106S–2122S.

Piwoz, E. 2004. *Nutrition and HIV/AIDS: Evidence, gaps and priority actions.* Washington, D.C.: Academy for Educational Development.

Piwoz, E., and E. Preble. 2000. *HIV/AIDS and nutrition: A review of the literature and recommendations for nutritional care and support in sub-Saharan Africa.* SARA Project. Washington, D.C.: U.S. Agency for International Development.

Polsky, B., D. Kotler, and C. Steinhart. 2004. Treatment guidelines for HIV-associated wasting. *HIV Clinical Trials* 5 (1): 50–61.

Poss, M., H. L. Martin, J. K. Kreiss, L. Granville, B. Chohan, P. Nyange, K. Mandaliya, and J. Overbaugh. 1995. Diversity in virus populations from genital secretions and peripheral blood from women recently infected with human immunodeficiency virus type 1. *Journal of Virology* 69 (12): 8118–8122.

Prins, M., R. P. Brettle, J. R. Robertson, I. Hernandez Aguado, B. Broers, N. Carre, et al. 1999. Geographical variation in disease progression in HIV-1 seroconverted injecting drug users in Europe. *International Journal of Epidemiology* 28: 541–549.

Reardon, T. 1997. Using evidence of household income diversification to inform study of the rural nonfarm labor market in Africa. *World Development* 25 (5): 735–748.

Reardon, T., C. Delgado, and P. Matlon. 1992. Determinants and effects of income diversification amongst farm households in Burkina Faso. *Journal of Development Studies* 28 (1): 264–296.

Remacha, A. F., J. Cadafalch, P. Sardà, M. Barceló, and M. Fuster. 2003. Vitamin B-12 metabolism in HIV-infected patients in the age of highly active antiretroviral therapy: Role of homocysteine in assessing vitamin B-12 status. *American Journal of Clinical Nutrition* 77 (2): 420–424.

Rosen, S., and J. L. Simon. 2002. Shifting the Burden of HIV/AIDS. Boston: Center for International Health, Boston University.

Ross, J. S., and M. H. Labbok. 2004. Modeling the effects of different infant feeding strategies on infant survival and mother to child transmission of HIV. *American Journal of Public Health* 94: 1174–1180.

Rottingen, J. A., D. W. Cameron, and G. P. Garnett. 2001. A systematic review of the epidemiologic interactions between classic sexually transmitted diseases and HIV: How much really is known? *Sexually Transmitted Diseases* 28 (10): 579–597.

Rousseau, M. C., C. Molines, J. Moreau, and J. Delmont. 2000. Influence of highly active antiretroviral therapy on micronutrient profiles in HIV-infected patients. *Annals of Nutrition and Metabolism* 44 (5–6): 212–216.

Roy, S. K., R. H. Behrens, R. Haider, S. M. Akramuzzaman, D. Mahalanabis, M. A. Wahed, and A. M. Tomkins. 1992. Impact of zinc supplementation on intestinal permeability in Bangladeshi children with acute diarrhoea and persistent diarrhoea syndrome. *Journal of Pediatrics Gastroenterology and Nutrition* 15 (3): 289–296.

Rugalema, G. 1999. Adult mortality as entitlement failure: AIDS and the crisis of rural livelihoods in a Tanzanian village. Ph.D. diss., Institute of Social Studies, The Hague.

———. 2000. Coping or struggling: A journey into the impact of HIV/AIDS in southern Africa. *Review of African Political Economy* 86: 537–545.

Rugalema, G., S. Weigang, and J. Mbwika. 1999. *HIV/AIDS and the commercial agricultural sector of Kenya: Impact, vulnerability, susceptibility and coping strategies.* Extension, Education and Communication Service (SDRE) and Research, Extension and Training (SDR) Division of FAO. Rome: FAO and UNDP.

Saag, M. S. 2004. Initiation of antiretroviral therapy: Implications of recent findings. *Topics in HIV Medicine* 12 (3): 83–88.

SADC FANR (Southern African Development Community Food, Agriculture, and Natural Resources Development Unit, Vulnerability Assessment Committee). 2003. *Towards identifying impacts of HIV/AIDS on food security in southern Africa and implications for response: Findings from Malawi, Zambia and Zimbabwe.* Harare, Zimbabwe.

Schwenk, A., A. Beisenherz, G. Kremer, V. Diehl, B. Salzberger, and G. Fätkenheuer. 1999. Bioelectrical impedance analysis in HIV-infected patients treated with triple antiretroviral treatment. *American Journal of Clinical Nutrition* 70 (5): 867–873.

Scott, G., and C. Harland. 2003. Food insecurity, HIV/AIDS and children. Washington, D.C.: Family Health International.

Scrimshaw, N., C. Taylor, and J. Gordon. 1968. *Interactions of nutrition and infection.* Geneva: World Health Organization.

Semba, R. D. 2000. Mastitis and transmission of human immunodeficiency virus through breast milk. *Annals of the New York Academy of Science* 918: 156–162.

Semba, R. D., and M. Neville. 1999. Breast-feeding, mastitis, and HIV transmission: Nutritional implications. *Nutrition Reviews* 5 (1): 146–153.

Semba, R. D., and A. M. Tang. 1999. Micronutrients and the pathogenesis of human immunodeficiency virus infection. *British Journal of Nutrition* 81 (3): 181–189.

Semba, R. D., J. D. Chiphangwi, P. G. Miotti, G. A. Dallabetta, D. Hoover, J. K. Canner, and A. Saah. 1994. Maternal vitamin A deficiency and mother-to-child transmission of HIV-1. *Lancet* 343: 1593–1597.

Semba, R. D., W. T. Caiaffa, N. M. Graham, S. Cohn, and D. Vlahov. 1995. Vitamin A deficiency and wasting as predictors of mortality in human immunodeficiency virus-infected injection drug users. *Journal of Infectious Diseases* 171 (5): 1196–1202.

Semba, R. D., P. G. Miotti, J. D. Chiphangwi, L. P. Yang, A. Saah, and D. Hoover. 1998. Maternal vitamin A deficiency and infant mortality in Malawi. *Journal of Tropical Pediatrics* 44 (4): 232–234.

Semba, R. D., N. Shah, and D. Vlahov. 2001. Improvement of anemia among HIV-infected injection drug users receiving highly active antiretroviral therapy. *Journal of Acquired Immune Deficiency Syndromes* 26 (4): 315–319.

Sen, A. 1981. *Poverty and famines: An essay on entitlement and deprivation.* Oxford: Clarendon Press.

Shah, M. K., N. Osborne, M. Mbilizi, and G. Vilili. 2001. *Impact of HIV/AIDS on agriculture productivity and rural livelihoods in the central region of Malawi.* Lilongwe, Malawi: Care International in Malawi.

Silva, M., P. R. Skolnik, S. L. Gorbach, et al. 1998. The effect of protease inhibitors on weight and body composition in HIV-infected patients. *AIDS* 12: 1645–1651.

Smith, L., and L. Haddad. 2000. *Explaining child malnutrition in developing countries: A cross-country analysis.* Research Report 111. Washington, D.C.: International Food Policy Research Institute.

Stillwaggon, E. 2000. HIV transmission in Latin America: Comparison with Africa and policy implications. *Journal of South African Economics* 48 (5): 985–1011.

———. 2002. HIV/AIDS in Africa: Fertile terrain. *Journal of Development Studies* 38 (6): 1–22.

Stokes, C. S. 2002. Measuring impacts of HIV/AIDS on rural livelihoods and food security. Rome: Gender and Population Division, FAO.

Strickland, R. 2004. *To have and to hold: Women's property and inheritance rights in the context of HIV/AIDS in sub-Saharan Africa.* Washington, D.C.: International

Center for Research on Women (ICRW) and the Global Coalition on Women and AIDS.

Suttmann, U., J. Ockenga, O. Selberg, L. Hoogestraat, H. Deicher, and M. J. Muller. 1995. Incidence and prognostic value of malnutrition and wasting in human immunodeficiency virus-infected outpatients. *Journal of Acquired Immune Deficiency Syndromes & Human Retrovirology* 8 (3): 239–246.

Tang, A. M. 2003. Weight loss, wasting, and survival in HIV-positive patients: Current strategies. *AIDS Reader* 13 (Supplement 12): S23–S27.

Tang, A. M., N. M. Graham, A. J. Kirby, L. D. McCall, W. C. Willett, and A. J. Saah. 1993. Dietary micronutrient intake and risk of progression to acquired immunodeficiency syndrome (AIDS) in human immunodeficiency virus type 1 (HIV-1)–infected homosexual men. *American Journal of Epidemiology* 138 (11): 937–951.

Tang, A. M., N. M. Graham, and A. J. Saah. 1996. Effects of micronutrient intake on survival in human immunodeficiency virus type 1 infection. *American Journal of Epidemiology* 143 (12): 1244–1256.

Tang, A. M., N. M. Graham, R. D. Semba, and A. J. Saah. 1997a. Association between serum vitamin A and E levels and HIV-1 disease progression. *AIDS* 11 (5): 613–620.

Tang, A. M., N. M. Graham, R. K. Chandra, and A. J. Saah. 1997b. Low serum vitamin B-12 concentrations are associated with faster human immunodeficiency virus type 1 (HIV-1) disease progression. *Journal of Nutrition* 127 (2): 345–351.

Tang, A. M., et al. 2002. Weight loss and survival in HIV-positive patients in the era of highly active antiretroviral therapy. *Journal of Acquired Immune Deficiency Syndromes* 31: 230–236.

TANGO International. 2002. *An initiative to address HIV/AIDS in the region.* Kampala, Uganda: East and Southern Africa Bureau, World Food Programme.

Thomas, K., S. P. Thyagarajan, L. Jaysellan, J. C. Varghese, P. Krishnamurthy, L. Bai, S. Hira, and K. Sudhakar. 2002. Community prevalence of sexually transmitted diseases and human immunodeficiency virus infection in Tamil Nadu, India: A probability proportional to size cluster survey. *National Medical Journal of India* 15 (3): 135–140.

Tibaijuka, A. K. 1997. AIDS and economic welfare in peasant agriculture: Case studies from Kagabiro village, Kagera region, Tanzania. *World Development* 25 (6): 963–975.

Tomkins, A. 2004. *Nutrition and HIV/AIDS Working Group of the SCN. A report of a meeting held at UNICEF, New York, 24 March 2004.* http://www.unsystem.org/scn.

Tomkins, A., and F. Watson. 1989. *Malnutrition and infection.* Geneva: ACC/SCN State-of-the-Art Series Nutrition Policy Discussion Paper 5.

Topouzis, D. 2003. *Addressing the impact of HIV/AIDS on ministries of agriculture: Focus on eastern and southern Africa.* Rome: FAO/UNAIDS.

UNAIDS. 1999. *Gender and HIV/AIDS: Taking stock of research and programs.* Geneva: UNAIDS Best Practice Collection. http://www.unaids.org/publications/documents/human/gender/una99e16.pdf.

———. 2004. Care, women and AIDS. Geneva.

UNAIDS/UNICEF. 2004. *The framework for protection, care and support of orphans and vulnerable children living in a world with HIV/AIDS.* Geneva.

UNAIDS/UNICEF/USAID. 2004. *Children on the brink: A joint report of new orphan estimates and a framework for action.* New York: UNICEF.

UNAIDS/UNICEF/WHO. 2004. *Epidemiological fact sheets on HIV/AIDS and sexually transmitted infections: India.* Geneva: UNAIDS.

UNAIDS/WHO 2004. *AIDS Epidemic Update.* Geneva.

UNAIDS/World Bank. 2001. AIDS, poverty reduction, and debt relief: A toolkit for mainstreaming HIV/AIDS programmes into development instruments. Geneva: UNAIDS Best Practice Collection.

UNDP. 2002. *HIV/AIDS and poverty reduction strategies: Policy note.* New York.

UNDP. 2003. *Human development report 2003. Millennium Development Goals: A compact among nations to end human poverty.* New York: Oxford University Press.

———. 2004. *Farmer's Life School Manual.* UNDP South East Asia HIV and Development Programme. Bangkok: UNDP/FAO and World Education.

United Nations. 2004. *Organizing the UN response to the triple threat of food insecurity, weakened capacity for governance and AIDS, particularly in southern and eastern Africa.* United Nations, New York.

Urassa, M., J. T. Boerma, Z. L. Japheth, J. Ng'weshemi, R. Isingo, D. Schapink, and Y. Kumogola. 1997. Orphanhood, child fostering and the AIDS epidemic in rural Tanzania. *Health Transition Review* 7 (Supplement 2): 141–153.

Urassa, M., J. T. Boerma, R. Isingo, J. Ngalula, J. Ng'weshemi, G. Mwaluko, and

B. Zaba. 2001. The impact of HIV/AIDS on mortality and household mobility in rural Tanzania. *AIDS* 15 (15): 2017–2023.

USAID. 2000. *AIDS Brief: Subsistence Agriculture Sector.* Washington, D.C.: USAID Africa Bureau.

Verweel, G., A. M. Van Rossum, N. G. Hartwig, T. F. Wolfs, H. J. Scherpbier, and R. de Groot. 2002. Treatment with highly active antiretroviral therapy in human immunodeficiency virus type 1–infected children is associated with a sustained effect on growth. *Pediatrics* 109 (2): E25–31.

Villamor, E., R. Mbise, D. Spiegelman, E. Hertzmark, M. Fataki, K. E. Peterson, G. Ndossi, and W. W. Fawzi. 2002. Vitamin A supplements ameliorate the adverse effect of HIV-1, malaria, and diarrheal infections on child growth. *Pediatrics* 109 (1): E6.

Wanke, C. A., M. Silva, T. A. Knox, J. Forrester, D. Spiegelman, and S. L. Gorbach. 2000. Weight loss and wasting remain common complications in individuals infected with human immunodeficiency virus in the era of highly active antiretroviral therapy. *Clinical Infectious Diseases* 31 (3): 803–805.

Weiser, S., W. Wolfe, D. Bangsberg, I. Thior, P. Gilbert, J. Makhema, P. Kebaabetswe, D. Dickenson, K. Mompati, M. Essex, and R. Marlink. 2003. Barriers to antiretroviral adherence for patients living with HIV infection and AIDS in Botswana. *Journal of Acquired Immune Deficiency Syndromes* 34 (3): 281–288.

WFP (World Food Programme). 2002. *Food and education: WFP's role in improving access to education for orphans and vulnerable children in sub-Saharan Africa.* Rome: Strategy and Policy Division, World Food Programme.

Wheeler, D. A., C. L. Gilbert, C. A. Launer, N. Muurahainen, R. A. Elion, D. I. Abrams, and G. E. Bartsch. 1998. Weight loss as a predictor of survival and disease progression in HIV infection. *Journal of Acquired Immune Deficiency Syndromes* 18 (1): 80–85.

White, J. 2002. *Facing the challenge: NGO experiences of mitigating the impacts of HIV/AIDS in sub-Saharan Africa.* London: Natural Resource Institute, University of Greenwich.

Whiteside, A., A. Hickey, A. Ngcobo, and J. Tomlinson. 2003. *What is driving the HIV/AIDS epidemic in Swaziland, and what more can we do about it?* Durban: National Emergency Response Committee on HIV/AIDS (NERCHA); UNAIDS; Health Economics and HIV/AIDS Research Division (HEARD).

WHO (World Health Organization). 2001. *New data on the prevention of mother-*

to-child transmission of HIV and their policy implications: Conclusions and recommendations. Geneva. www.unaids.org/publications/documents/mtct.

———. 2002. *Scaling up antiretroviral therapy in resource limited settings: Guidelines for a public health approach.* Geneva.

———. 2003. *Nutrient requirements for people living with HIV/AIDS: Report of a technical consultation.* Geneva.

Wisner, B., P. Blaikie, T. Cannon, and I. Davis. 2004. *At risk: Natural hazards, people's vulnerability and disasters.* 2nd ed. London: Routledge.

World Bank. 1993. *Sexually transmitted infections: Prevention and care project, Zimbabwe.* Staff Appraisal Report 11730-ZIM. Washington, D.C.

———. 2002. *World Development Indicators 2002.* CD-ROM. Washington, D.C.

Yamano, T., and T. S. Jayne. 2004. Measuring the impact of working-age adult mortality on small-scale farm households in Kenya. *World Development* 32 (1): 91–119.

———. Forthcoming. Working-age adult mortality and primary school attendance in rural Kenya. *Economic Development and Cultural Change.*

Yeh, K. C., P. J. Deutsch, H. Haddix, M. Hesney, V. Hoagland, W. D. Ju, S. J. Justice, B. Osborne, A. T. Sterrett, J. A. Stone, E. Woolf, and S. Waldman. 1998. Single-dose pharmacokinetics of indinavir and the effect of food. *Antimicrobial Agents and Chemotherapy* 42 (2): 332–338.

Zachariah, R., M. P. Spielmann, A. D. Harries, and F. M. Salaniponi. 2002. Moderate to severe malnutrition in patients with tuberculosis is a risk factor associated with early death. *Transactions of the Royal Society for Tropical Medicine and Hygiene* 96 (3): 291–294.

Zambia VAC (Vulnerability Assessment Committee) and SADC FANR VAC. 2003. *Zambia VAC April 2003 livelihood and vulnerability assessment.* Lusaka, Zambia.

Zuma, K., E. Gouws, B. Williams, and M. Lurie. 2003. Risk factors for HIV infection among women in Carletonville, South Africa: Migration, demography and sexually transmitted diseases. *International Journal of STD & AIDS* 14 (12): 814–817.

Stuart Gillespie is a senior research fellow in IFPRI's Food Consumption and Nutrition Division (FCND) and cofounder and director of RENEWAL, the Regional Network on HIV/AIDS, Rural Livelihoods and Food Security.

Suneetha Kadiyala is a research analyst in FCND.

Made in the USA
Monee, IL
13 September 2026

62981019R00105